WOMEN'S HEALTH COUNTS

In the current climate of medical audit, cost effectiveness, and the selective use of statistics for political purposes no one concerned with women's health can afford to dismiss what can be learned through the use of statistics.

While a women-centred approach to health has traditionally been seen as relying on women's own experiences and accounts, there is an important place for the effective use and analysis of hard data in studies of women's health and illness.

This collection is an introduction to the main sources of statistical data and illustrates the problems which may arise from their collection and use.

Women's Health Counts also explores the extent and limitations of official data: shows what can be learned from large data sets; presents some of the issues of concern in the use of randomized controlled trials, and looks at the way in which qualitative research may help us interpret statistical data, as well as placing the use of quantitative data on women and health in its political and social context.

WOMEN'S HEALTH COUNTS

edited by
HELEN ROBERTS

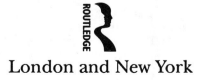

London and New York

First published 1990
by Routledge
11 New Fetter Lane, London EC4P 4EE

Simultaneously published in the USA and Canada
by Routledge
a division of Routledge, Chapman and Hall, Inc.
29 West 35th Street, New York, NY 10001

Typeset by LaserScript Ltd, Mitcham, Surrey
Printed and bound in Great Britain by
Biddles Ltd, Guildford and King's Lynn

British Library Cataloguing in Publication Data
Women's health counts.
1. Women. Health. Sociological perspectives.
I. Roberts, Helen, *1949–*
305.4

Library of Congress Cataloging in Publication Data
Women's health counts / Helen Roberts (editor).
p.   cm.
Statistical data reproduced from various sources.
Includes bibliographical references.
1. Women – Health and hygiene – Statistical methods.
2. Women – Medical care – Statistical methods.   3. Health surveys.
I. Roberts, Helen, 1949–   .
[DNLM: 1. Data Interpretation, Statistical.
2. Health Surveys – Great Britain – statistics.   3. Women – Great
Britain – statistics.   WA 900 FA1 W8]
RA564.85W674   1990
613'.04244'072–dc20
DNLM/DLC for Library of Congress
89–70188
CIP

ISBN 0-415-04890-7

CONTENTS

CONTENTS

CONTRIBUTORS

Sara Arber is Senior Lecturer in Sociology, University of Surrey, teaching mainly research methodology and medical sociology. She was a Member of the ESRC Social Affairs Committee, 1984–7, the ESRC Working Group on the 1991 Census, 1987 to present, and Treasurer of the British Sociological Association, 1988–90. Her current research is on carers and the elderly. Her publications include A. Dale, S. Arber, and M. Procter (1988) *Doing Secondary Analysis*, a series of teaching data sets: *Exploring British Society*, and numerous articles.

Hilary Graham is Professor of Applied Social Studies at the University of Warwick. She has worked previously at the Universities of York and Bradford, at the Open University and at Coventry Polytechnic. Her research on women's health has centred on women's experiences of caring in poverty, looking in particular at how women – in both one- and two-parent households – cope with caring for young children. Women's smoking in the context of both poverty and caring has been a continuing focus of her research.

Alison Macfarlane worked as a statistician on a variety of subjects, including animal husbandry, traffic surveys, air pollution, and child health before she joined the National Perinatal Epidemiology Unit soon after it was first set up in 1978. She has worked there since, specializing in the analyses of routinely collected statistics about the maternity services and the people who use them.

Claudia Martin is a Senior Research Fellow at the Local Government Centre, University of Warwick, where she is working on inter-agency strategies to combat poverty. Previously, she was at the Research Unit in Health and Behavioural Change, University of Edinburgh, where her main area of research concerned the effects of housing conditions and unemployment on child health.

Kath Moser was until recently a research fellow at the Social Statistics Research Unit at City University where she has been doing research on inequalities in health using data from the OPCS Longitudinal Study. Her particular areas of interest have been women's mortality, and also the relationship between unemployment and mortality.

Ann Oakley is a sociologist, researcher, and writer. She is currently Deputy Director at the Thomas Coram Research Unit in London, working on research concerning the health of women and young people. She has published a number of books on the position of women, the family and health issues, and, more recently, a novel.

Helena Pugh was until recently a research fellow at the Social Statistics Research Unit at City University, working on a project concerned with inequalities in health. In particular, her interests include measuring differences in women's mortality and the relationship between social class and specific causes of death. She has also carried out research on female secretarial and clerical homeworkers. She now works as a local government research officer.

Helen Roberts is a medical sociologist with the Social Paediatric and Obstetric Research Unit in Glasgow. Her previous work includes *Doing Feminist Research* (1981), *The Patient Patients* (1985), and (with Ann Oakley and Ann McPherson) *Miscarriage* (1990). She has developed a social classification scheme for women on the basis of data from the Longitudinal Study, and is currently working on disadvantage and child health, the epidemiology of ectopic pregnancy in Scotland, and miscarriage.

Philip Y. K. Teo is a Senior Registrar in Public Health Medicine with the Greater Glasgow Health Board and a Research Fellow with the Social Paediatric and Obstetric Research Unit, University of Glasgow. His research interests are health care evaluation and various aspects of maternal and child health.

ACKNOWLEDGEMENTS

There are many contributors to the making of a book whose names do not appear on the contents page. Some of those involved in producing this book are acknowledged in individual chapters. As editor, my own particular debts are to Margaret Appleton, Rodney Barker, and David Stone for intellectual and practical help, to John Fox and my former colleagues at the Social Statistics Research Unit, City University, for teaching me about large data sets, and to the contributors to this volume. At Routledge, Gill Davies, Caroline Lane and Jo Thurm have been most helpful. It was a pleasure to be able to work with them.

The following are gratefully acknowledged for permission to reproduce tables: the Office of Population Censuses and Surveys for data in chapter 4. OPCS gave permission for the use of the General Household Survey data described in chapter 3 and the ESRC data archive at the University of Essex supplied the data. Data used in chapter 5 were supplied by the Information and Statistics Division of the Common Services Agency of the Scottish Health Service and the data for England and Wales used in Figure 5.1 was provided through an ad hoc data request to OPCS. The original version of chapter 7 was published in the journal *Women and Health* (Oakley 1990) and we are most grateful to the editors and publishers for permission to reproduce it here. For tables in chapter 8, some of which are recalculations, the authors and sources are warmly acknowledged, as are the King's Fund for permission to reproduce Table 8.2, the Health Promotion Research Trust for permission to reproduce Tables 8.4, 8.5, 8.6, and 8.8, and the Gower Publishing Group for permission to reproduce Table 8.7, and the Family Studies Centre for permissions in relation to Table 8.9. Crown copyright is reserved on chapters 2 and 4. Karen Dunnell and Isobel Macdonald Davies at OPCS have been particularly helpful in responding to queries concerning permissions.

All of us owe a more general debt to women who contribute their experience to researchers, to those who collect and analyse data which enable researchers to look at the social determinants of women's health and illness, and to those who use these data well.

Chapter One

WOMEN'S HEALTH COUNTS

HELEN ROBERTS

In recent years, and to some extent in response to the women's movement, there has been an upsurge of interest in research on women's health. That this is not merely an 'academic' matter can be seen in the extent to which the press, ranging from the tabloids to the heavier dailies, covers health issues and health research. Work on health is, of course, of more than academic interest to all of us, an observation encapsulated in the title of the worldwide bestseller produced by the Boston women's health collective, *Our Bodies Ourselves* (Boston Women's Health Book Collective 1978).

The collection of essays in this book presents a range of writing on hard data concerning women's health and is aimed at users and providers of health research. It proceeds on the assumption that, particularly in view of the current political preoccupation with audit and 'cost effectiveness' in health, a good understanding of the range, use, and possibilities of statistics on women's health is an important part of our education.

THE AIMS AND SCOPE OF THE COLLECTION

The primary aim of this collection is to serve as an introduction to some of the main sources of statistical data on women's health and illness, to look at some of the problems which may arise in their collection and use, to give a series of examples which demonstrate what can be done in terms of analysis, and to look at some of the difficulties involved in quantitative research on women's health.

An aversion to looking at figures or to understanding how they may be analysed and used is not helpful in the current climate. One introductory paperback on the (mis)use of statistics is beguilingly entitled: *How to Lie with Statistics* (Huff 1973). In many cases, there would be little need for those producing statistics to lie, as the eye of the reader glances over sets of statistics to get to the text and the interpretative material. But those who deal with statistics are not, as their detractors would have it, mere 'number crunchers'. No advertising agency, employed to demonstrate the creative as well as the scientific skills of statisticians, could have come up with a better line than the cartoonist Mel Calman's contribution to the inside cover of *How to Lie with Statistics*: 'Don't be a novelist – be a statistician. Much more scope for the imagination'. While this tongue-in-cheek comment was no doubt intended to draw attention to the statistical 'tricks' so ably outlined by Huff, the authors of the following chapters amply demonstrate the importance of the use of the imagination as well as the intellect in generating, understanding, and analysing data.

While this is not a textbook in content, construction, or style, there is a certain didactic intent. Each of the chapters sets out, though in different ways, to show what can be done with quantitative data. First, in Alison Macfarlane's chapter, we are given some background to the history of the collection of statistical data on health and illness. The main data sources open to those who might want to do research on women's health are described and critically appraised. What data are available on women and health? What do they tell us (and what do they not tell us)? What are their strengths and weaknesses? And how might they be improved? Statistics are, of course, a social construct, and have to be understood within the context in which they are generated, collected, analysed, and interpreted. Alison Macfarlane's own work contains numerous examples of the careful analysis and interpretation of statistics on maternal and child health, and she has the skill of presenting her work to a variety of different readerships and audiences (Macfarlane 1988a, 1988b; Macfarlane and Mugford 1984; Campbell and Macfarlane 1987). This is important, because part of the power of official and other statistics lies in the fact that there tends to be a rather restricted readership, with much of the material directed towards the *cognoscenti* of epidemiological and statistical data. Access to quantitative data may be seen as privileged. As Irvine *et al.* (1979: 2) write in their introduction to *Demystifying Social Statistics*: 'Quantitative knowledge is . . . set apart from all other forms of social knowledge: statistical data are held to be objective, whereas qualitative data are much more likely to be seen as ideological', but they point out that 'The total rejection of statistics is as one-sided as an uncritical acceptance of all that statistics orthodoxy tells us – both discourage critical scrutiny of the important part played by statistics and the social context in which they have developed' (ibid).

This is the starting point for Alison Macfarlane's chapter, where she draws attention to the historical background to the collection of official statistics, the main sources of official statistics, and data specifically collected on women. She gives examples of ways in which statistics may be misinterpreted, and makes clear the way in which the purpose for which they are originally collected can restrict what we can learn from the data. She looks at the strengths and shortcomings of official statistics on women's health and illness, but is realistic about change. As she herself has written: 'fundamental improvements in medical statistics are unlikely to occur in the absence of changes in the prevailing view of the nature of health and the causes of illness. To paraphrase a well known saying: official statisticians have enumerated society. The point is to change it' (Macfarlane 1980: 60).

The three chapters which follow are based on particular large-scale data sets. Sara Arber's chapter draws on the General Household Survey (GHS), Helena Pugh and Kath Moser draw on the Office of Population Censuses and Surveys Longitudinal Study (LS), and Philip Teo's chapter is based on the Scottish Morbidity Record (SMR). In each of these, examples are given of what can be (and what has been) done with the data in terms of particular problems. What can the GHS tell us about women's sickness absence? What can we learn from the GHS about the care of the elderly in their own homes? Is it in fact daughters who do most of the work in caring for the frail elderly? How can the GHS be used to throw light on the problem of using women's social class as a means of understanding inequalities in health? Some ways in which analysis of survey data can be used to answer these and other practical questions are given in Sara Arber's chapter on 'Using the General Household Survey to Analyse Women's Health'. Although, as Alison Macfarlane explains in her chapter, there are a number of respects in which routinely collected data in relation to women's health are deficient, it is also the case that there is a great deal of rich data which is underused. A government social survey is a highly professional exercise, producing survey material which would be difficult to replicate in terms of quality or quantity by the average researcher. Sara Arber, who with her colleagues at the University of Surrey has done a great deal of work in opening up this data base to researchers, describes the practicalities of accessing data from the General Household Survey. She goes on to illustrate through three case-studies, based on her work with colleagues, the ways in which these data may be used to provide an answer to both practical and intellectual questions on women's health. Do women have a higher rate of sickness absence than men, and are insurance companies justified in charging a higher premium for permanent health insurance for women than for men? While her first example refutes a myth about women's sickness absence, her second example, looking at gender differences and the care of the elderly, reveals that the widely held view that care of the elderly in the home is provided almost entirely by women is mistaken. While Arber and her colleagues have been able to show the disadvantaged position of married women with regard to the provision of services to elderly people with whom they are co-resident, they also show that about 40 per cent of carers of the frail elderly are men. Finally, addressing the important issue of social class and inequality in health, which is also the focus of chapters by Hilary Graham and Helena Pugh and Kath Moser, Arber looks at the way in which women's social class can be re-analysed on the basis of GHS data and related to health status data provided from the same source.

Other researchers can use this under-analysed data set, as Arber makes clear. The main reasons they might want to do so are the quality of the data and, as Arber shows, the extent of the insights which can be provided from the analysis. But perhaps in the current climate the fact that the use of these high quality data is extremely cost-effective provides a further impetus. Secondary analysis cuts out some of the costs of other sorts of research.

In addition to the General Household Survey, a number of other government and non-government social surveys collect data which can be used to look at women's health. An excellent source book for these is Ann Cartwright's *Health Surveys* (1983) which has a good breadth of coverage although it is not, of course, restricted to women's health.

What of large-scale data which is not collected through surveys, and its use for the study of inequalities in women's health? This is addressed in the chapter by Helena Pugh and Kath Moser. While Arber concentrates on women's morbidity, Pugh and Moser look at women's mortality. They use the information from an important large data set, the Office of Population Censuses and Surveys Longitudinal Study (LS) to construct a new way of measuring differences in women's mortality. The LS comprises a 1 per cent sample of the population of England and Wales from the 1971 census drawn up by using four dates of birth. This was followed up in 1981 and there are plans for follow-up in 1991 via census information. Census records for sample members have been linked with information on subsequent events about which details are routinely collected, including live and stillbirths to sample members, deaths of sample members and their spouses, and cancer registrations. The sample is kept up to date by the addition of new births and immigrants and the removal of LS members who have died or emigrated. The Longitudinal Study has many strengths. As Marsh (1988) writes, 'the survey is already considered to be one of the most important databases for the study of mortality, fertility and mobility available to researchers, and its value increases as the years go by'.

The first programme of work on the LS concentrated on mortality, and looked at the complex relationships between mortality and a range of characteristics including economic activity, social class, household structure, marital status, and marital and fertility history. More recently, the early work on the relationship between female mortality and social circumstances has been developed and is described in the chapter by Helena Pugh and Kath Moser. Situating their discussion within the context of the inequalities in health debate, they use data from the LS to examine women's mortality. Developing the point made by Alison Macfarlane on the difficulties of using conventional social class measures to classify women adequately, they use a broader classification, more appropriate to women's lives, to look at deaths of women aged 15–59 during the period 1976–81. Using a combination of household variables, such as housing tenure and access to a car, alongside occupational information to differentiate more finely between large groups of women, and using standard-ized mortality ratios (SMRs) as a summary index of mortality, they

5

demonstrate how widely the mortality of women in England and Wales varies according to their social circumstances. A strength of this chapter is that it presents a potential way forward for any study planning to group women using some sort of social classification. As the authors point out, much of the information required for this alternative approach is already collected. It is simply a matter of making full use of existing data.

There is a rather different unique data set of use to health researchers in Scotland. This is the Scottish Morbidity Record which is a rich database with a high level of reliability and validity covering all episodes of in-patient hospital treatment in NHS hospitals in Scotland.

There are a number of areas where rising levels of surgical intervention in relation to women have caused concern. One such operation is caesarian section, another hysterectomy – both are major operations. The indications, or reasons for doing these operations, have broadened, and in many cases there is lack of consensus over whether the operation was strictly necessary. Recent concern by feminists was pre-dated by some years in an article by a male physician published in 1946 entitled 'Hysterectomy: therapeutic necessity or surgical racket?' (Miller 1946). A gift to those critical of rising levels of hysterectomy has been Wright's much quoted editorial in which he claimed that 'After the last planned pregnancy, the uterus becomes a useless, bleeding, symptom producing, potentially cancer bearing organ and should be removed' (Wright 1969). But is this view not anachronistic? Perhaps not. Some twenty years on, in an editorial in the *British Journal of Obstetrics and Gynaecology* on the prophylactic removal of the ovaries (oophorectomy) John Studd concludes: 'Prophylactic oophorectomy should be offered to all women over the age of 40 having an abdominal hysterectomy but should only be performed after adequate discussion, understanding and of course consent. The woman has the ultimate choice. If she exercises what is perhaps the only worthwhile argument against prophylactic oophorectomy, *namely a sentimental desire to keep her ovaries* [my emphasis], then it would be a foolish and insensitive gynaecologist who ignores this compelling argument' (Studd 1989: 508). One could only speculate on whether a similar attachment of a male to his testes after his fathering days were over would be seen as purely sentimental, perhaps irrational, in view of the testicular cancer to which he might be exposing himself by their retention.

There have been a number of good studies based on data from England and Wales on rising rates of hysterectomy (McPherson *et al.* 1981; Coulter and McPherson 1986; Coulter *et al.* 1988). Until now, the only published Scottish work, at a time when there has been a steep rise in the rate of hysterectomy in NHS hospitals in Scotland, has been a regional study (Grant and Hussein 1984). Philip Teo's chapter looks more closely at some of the statistics behind hysterectomy on the basis of his study of hysterectomy over the period 1961–84. Teo's chapter is based on the routine collection of hospital in-patient data in Scotland. He uses these data to look at the steep rise in the rate of hysterectomy in Scotland, describes what the components of this rise are, and offers a range of speculative explanations based on these data. He examines the question of whether the rate of hysterectomy has risen to meet the number of gynaecologists available, what the regional variations are, and what the lifetime chances are of a woman in Scotland having a hysterectomy. He shows how the data can be used to look at trends over time, including trends by age groups. In this context, he is able to show how the 'blips' in the data at the time of trade union action, when the rate of hysterectomy dropped, differentially affected different age groups. He looks at changes in diagnostic indications (reasons) for the operation, changes in waiting time, changes in length of stay, and a variety of other data, including regional variations. He describes in some detail the particular data source he uses and its strengths and weaknesses and addresses some of the practical problems faced by the epidemiologist, such as the use of an appropriate denominator.

Following these chapters which deal with the secondary use of large-scale data sets, Claudia Martin discusses the problem from the point of view of an originator of a more modest set of data, describing the work that she and her colleagues did when they were asked to provide information which it was hoped might guide policy makers on their decisions on maternity care provision. Just as Teo's chapter examines the question of whether there are too many (or too few) hysterectomies, Martin's chapter too looks at the question of provision, but from another starting point. In 1986 the Health Board in Lothian, the area which includes Edinburgh, was faced with a number of decisions concerning the provision of maternity services. It was likely that at least one hospital would be closed. There was dismay among some of the users of maternity services, and Claudia Martin and her colleagues were commissioned to produce a report. The Health Board, it was felt, would be most likely to take cognizance of 'hard data'. Martin describes how she and her colleagues went about their work, how they constituted a sample, how they collected data, how these data were analysed, what the findings were, and how those findings were interpreted and used. There were, of course, considerable practical difficulties in collecting fairly large-scale, ad hoc data quickly for policy-making purposes. Martin's team was able to deliver on time, but their speed and efficiency, as she makes clear, was a double-edged sword.

It must be remembered that statistical data can be interpreted in a number of different ways and Martin explains different possible interpretations of the same data. She also looks at those who expressed dissatisfaction with existing services. While those in authority may congratulate themselves or heave a sigh of relief when these numbers are small, current political ideology makes customers of us all, and dissatisfied customers must have their needs addressed. Martin's chapter looks at the question of the use to which the survey was put. Cartwright (1983: 178) crisply remarks that 'researchers should be sensitive to the possibility that they might be asked to do a survey in order to reduce pressure for action or to postpone uncomfortable decisions'. Martin and her colleagues were indeed sensitive to this issue, although they were asked to do the work by users, rather than providers, of a service. But as Martin makes clear, carrying out a survey in this situation had political ramifications. Cartwright (1983) makes the important distinction between ethical and political decisions, pointing out that ethical ones relate to what is right or wrong, political ones to expediency and what is likely to happen. 'When we are anxious about the use of survey results I think these are political anxieties even though they may be about the unethical use of results' (Cartwright 1983: 178). While there is an extent to which Claudia Martin's chapter provides a cautionary tale on the generation of data on 'consumer' satisfaction, she describes some entirely satisfactory outcomes of the research. If satisfaction among users is to be improved and the quality of care monitored, it is clear that a mechanism is needed to know just what these views are. It cannot be assumed that the views of health service users can be adequately represented by the views of professionals and managers within the NHS, however well intentioned they may be.

Others who wish to carry out a consumer survey may be helped by a manual published by OPCS (Mason 1989) which describes how to carry out local surveys of users' views on maternity care. The manual describes how to carry out antenatal and postnatal surveys and points to the high level of response that can be expected from postal questionnaires in this area. The desire of women to make their feelings known can be judged by the fact that response rates averaging 75 per cent can be expected. In line with this, Martin and her colleagues had a response rate of 79 per cent, and we need to bear in mind that these were women recently delivered and caring for a baby who was just a few weeks old. If the motivation of women to make their feelings known is as high as this, there is an equally high responsibility on researchers to make the best use, interpretation, and analysis of these data.

Moving away from the collection and use of statistical data as such, the chapter by Ann Oakley, while dealing (like the other work in this book) with hard data, adopts a rather different approach by examining some of the problems of randomized controlled trials (RCTs). The RCT, which is sometimes seen as the major scientific means of evaluating medical research, is a test or 'trial' of a particular treatment or approach. It compares two or more groups of subjects who are allocated to these groups at random, that is, according to chance. One of the criticisms of clinical trials in the past, and particularly trials intended to look at the effectiveness of various treatments for cancer, is that they have tended to measure length of life, rather than quality of life after an intervention. As one patient wrote after a radical mastectomy: 'the rate of survival may look good in the statistics, but statistics don't count the cost' (quoted in Gore 1988). Sheila Gore has suggested that they can and should (Gore 1988). Indeed there have been a number of RCTs in the area of childbirth where one of the variables considered has been maternal satisfaction (for example, Flint and Poulengeris 1987). Using a number of examples, including the RCT of which she was a Director, Ann Oakley examines areas of conflict between feminist research and randomized controlled evaluation. She then discusses the general ethical issues of consent, certainty and uncertainty, and addresses the problem of random allocation in health research, using her own RCT of social support in pregnancy as an example.

Some of these issues have also been raised by patients. Evelyn Thomas participated in two randomized clinical trials without her knowledge or consent. She wrote later: 'Withholding information about the trials may have invalidated them. It was forgotten that patients, unlike laboratory animals, can move around and communicate with each other. Treatments are discussed and unexplained differences discovered. Inevitably, these cause worry, and patients may become confused and resentful. Such feelings, and the stress produced, may be the very factors which affect health and well being.' She added that as a scientist herself: 'I am not arguing against . . . RCTs. As a patient, I have the most to gain from progress . . . . But RCTs must only be used with the informed consent of the participating patients. If investigators cannot convince patients that each arm of an RCT carries an equal chance of risks or benefits, then they must respect those patients' decisions not to participate' (Thomas 1988). A charter of patients' rights in clinical research has recently been proposed in *The Lancet* (Herxheimer 1988). A number of the proposals accord with the arguments in Oakley's chapter and would meet the points raised so cogently by Evelyn Thomas.

The major part of this book is concerned with the use of quantitative data. It is perhaps appropriate that the final chapter should be based on methods which draw together the best of both qualitative and quantitative understanding. Hilary Graham's chapter demonstrates how a variety of large-scale and small-scale data sets, together with qualitative data, can be used to understand and explain health issues. It shows the importance of the intervention of the human intellect between the collection of data and their understanding. Graham's chapter is a good example of the imaginative synthesis of quantitative and qualitative methods, and demonstrates the importance of interpreting data within their social context. Very frequently, and quite properly, quantitative data will be used for descriptive purposes. In a sense, the data will be left to speak for themselves. If there is an established link between smoking and deaths from lung cancer and coronary heart disease, and if statistics reliably show that more working-class than middle-class women smoke, it would appear at first sight that the health message to be taken from this is a simple one. Hilary Graham successfully shows how these data should be our starting point rather than our end point, and that it is intelligent and imaginative interpretation which is the most useful tool in trying to understand the meaning of good quantitative data.

On the quantitative side, starting with a mortality table from OPCS, Graham sets out the main causes of death among women. She then turns to two sets of epidemiological work which suggest the risk factors behind these causes of death. Using another data set, the Health and Lifestyle Survey, she examines health-related behaviour among women. Who smokes? Who eats 'brown' bread? Who eats fruit regularly? Turning to women as paid and unpaid workers, both inside and outside the home, and including the important work of health maintenance routinely carried out by many women, she examines data from *British Social Attitudes* on the domestic division of labour. Returning to *The Health and Lifestyle Survey*, she uses their data to demonstrate that women's own assessments of the causes of ill health are far from being at variance with popularly promoted views on personal account-ability. Finally, and tellingly, she uses data from a Family Policy Studies Centre publication to illustrate the absolute and relative amounts spent by 'average' families and those on supplementary benefit on a variety of household goods and services.

Graham adds to this hard data qualitative data taken from her own and other scholars' interviews with women. For while the surveys provide data which could not economically be gathered in other ways, interviews by skilled researchers can contextualize the larger-scale findings. They provide an understanding of data which might otherwise appear baffling at best, and which at worst might lead to a cynical interpretation of the behaviour of those whom Graham rightly identifies as 'health keepers' but who nevertheless spend a sizeable proportion of their budget on tobacco.

Hilary Graham uses these data to weave an argument which illustrates the difference between two sorts of 'explanation' for health differences: the cultural/behavioural and the ma-terial/structural perspectives. But this is no mere academic exercise. If health promotion campaigns are to be effective (or in today's climate, perhaps the more appropriate term is *cost* effective) the implications of Graham's argument need to be

11

understood and implemented. If her interpretation is correct, slick phrases, such as that of 'making the healthy choice and the easy choice', are not merely misguided, but when operationalized, may have the reverse of the intended effect.

Iain Chalmers (Chalmers 1983) has suggested that one of the features of scientific enquiry is its anti-authoritarian nature. This is not perhaps the first feature of the scientific enterprise which might strike one. But Hilary Graham's chapter illustrates very well the way in which her active promotion of the scientific notions of uncertainty and enquiry, carefully pursued, can lead to new insights on topics such as smoking and health where it is 'self-evident' that smoking is bad for everybody's health.

SOURCES OF HELP IN THE HANDLING OF AND PRESENTATION OF STATISTICAL DATA

The material in this collection is presented so as to be quite within the grasp of those with no training in epidemiology, demography, statistics, or the handling of large-scale data. The text provides full explanation of the figures and tables accompanying each chapter. Those interested in the development of health statistics would do well to read Muriel Nissel's fascinating history of the General Register Office, *People Count* (Nissel 1987), which devotes two chapters to the development of health statistics. But for the reader or researcher with little background in data handling, who would like to know more, Catherine Marsh's book *Exploring Data: An Introduction to Data Analysis for Social Scientists* (Marsh 1988) is a good practical start, well presented, and with a number of exercises. Excellent discussions of the use social scientists can make of government statistics are also provided by Dale *et al.* (1988). For those looking for some background in medical statistics, Bland (1987) and Gore and Altman (1982) provide a good grounding. For advice on the presentation of data, or indeed as an aid to critically reading the studies of others, it is worthwhile to read the statistical guidelines for contributors to medical journals published by Altman *et al.* (1983) and the HMSO publication *Plain Figures* (Chapman with Mahon 1986).

THE AUTHORITY OF QUANTITATIVE DATA

On the one hand statistics may be viewed as tedious, on the other as untrustworthy. But the widespread distrust of statistics does not exorcise either the figures or the policies which they inspire, inform, or justify. We need to understand what statistics can and cannot tell us about health, as about anything else. An over-reverent approach to figures supports the empiricist fallacy that figures are merely given objective facts, a proper understanding of which compels one conclusion and one only. An over-sceptical approach sustains the equally erroneous belief that statistics are mere mystification, a way of obscuring truth and legitimizing error, that they are born in deception and formed of quantified ideology. Both of these approaches are misleading. Without evaluation and interpretation, numbers are inert. Statistics are not merely given life by thought, they are also a product of it. They are to that extent neither possessed of unquestionable objective authority, nor matters of mere fancy. They need to be handled with the same critical and imaginative care as is given to any other set of data or explanations.

That statistics are a social product can be illustrated by looking at some aspects of the recent history of the collection and publication of official statistics in the United Kingdom. Since 1979, there has been a reduction in the amount of published official statistics which has caused some disquiet to social scientists and other users. There have been changes in the way in which unemployment is measured, and the Decennial Supplement on Occupational Mortality published in 1986 gave tables for the first time in microfiche form (OPCS 1986a). This might be viewed as a welcome use of new technology, but one of the results was that the data were accessible only to those with a fiche reader. At the same time, there has been a steep rise in the cost of statistical publications. Some of these issues were taken up in a *British Medical Journal* (BMJ) editorial in 1986, entitled, 'Lies, Damned Lies and Suppressed Statistics'. The author asked what might be concluded from the absence in the Decennial Supplement of any attempt to analyse morbidity and mortality by social class, and suggested that 'potentially adverse information' was being suppressed. It is worth rehearsing some of the arguments which the author offered to support this view as attention is drawn to a number of the biases which may affect not only the collection and publication of statistics but also their entry into the public domain through, for instance, press reports. One example given in the editorial refers to changes in the definition of unemployment in recent years, all of which have served to reduce the total. Another example is taken from *Social Trends*, the admirably clear summary compendium of various aspects of official social statistics published annually. 'The 1986 edition of *Social Trends* compared the amount spent on housing by owner-occupiers and tenants, and showed the cost to owner-occupiers before tax relief and the cost to tenants after rebates had been deducted. The figures are thus not comparable, and exaggerate the amount that owner-occupiers pay' (*BMJ* 1986: 350). Other examples given of bias included the removal of a table on unemployment and health from *Social Trends* because there was no table on the health of those in employment, and a decision 'on economic grounds' to publish data on families living in poverty every two years rather than every year. On the point of the entry of data into the public domain, it was pointed out that when data were published showing an increase in the number of families living on supplementary benefit, 'they were "published" on the day that the House of Commons rose for the summer recess. They were placed in the library minutes before it closed' (p. 350). There was a similar problem when the 'Black Report' on inequalities in health, commissioned by a Labour administration but reporting to a Conservative Government, was published in the form of 260 typescripts on a Bank Holiday Monday. A follow-up report, commissioned by the (then) Health Education Council, but reporting to the re-named Health Education Authority, in 1987 had its press launch at the Health Education Authority cancelled at the last moment. Journalists were hastily re-directed to a back room at the premises of the nearby Disability Alliance where Sir Douglas Black, one of the authors of the original report, and present for the launch of the follow-up, no doubt had a sense of *déjà vu*.

Lest it be thought that the desire to keep potentially embarrassing data quiet is new, it is worth quoting from a memorandum from a civil servant referred to by Laurance (1986). This memorandum was written in 1976, that is, under a Labour rather than a Conservative government, and refers to deaths from hypothermia: 'In this politically sensitive area it is of great importance not to issue information which may be misleading and will

14

certainly be used against the government. Any reply suggesting large numbers of old people are suffering from hypothermia could be used to put pressure on the government to increase heating provision' (Laurance 1986: 350). In fairness, it should be pointed out that the (then) chief medical statistician at OPCS, Michael Alderson, disagreed with many of the claims made in the leading article in the *British Medical Journal.* He pointed out that the time lag from collection to publication of the Decennial Supplement had been halved, and made clear that '. . . users of the material may draw their own conclusions in relation to specific issues. We are always willing to help users of the material' (Alderson 1986: 503). Those of us who have contact through our work with researchers in OPCS can testify to the most helpful way in which requests for data and information are dealt with. Whether this can or should replace the ready entry of, for instance, social class mortality data directly into the public arena is a different matter.

What an examination of the use, presentation, and discussion of such public and official statistics shows is the authority of statistics. They are recognized to carry weight, and it is important for all those who wish to carry opinion with them to ensure that the oracle speaks in tones favourable to their own case. The presentation, publication, delay, or suppression of statistics are thus matters of more than merely academic significance. When the (then) Minister for the Environment, Nicholas Ridley, complained in the summer of 1989 that 'great confusion' was caused if 'wild accusations of this or that threat are treated as of no less validity than the official figures of those who painstakingly and honestly compile them' (*Scotsman* 1989) he was asserting his government's claim to the authoritative dispensation of incontestable information. Max Weber described governments as institutions successfully claiming the monopoly of legitimate coercion (Weber 1919: 78). But today they have the further characteristic of contesting for the monopoly of legitimate statistics. One function of such a use of statistics is to foreclose discussion, rather than to stimulate it.

QUALITATIVE AND QUANTITATIVE RESEARCH

This collection is based entirely around hard data, a form of information which feminists have often regarded with suspicion.

To some extent, the concentration in this volume on hard data is a deviation from the common assumption (mistaken in my view) that research by, for, or acceptable to feminists should be based on 'soft' methods – 'telling it like it is'. This view may well have its roots in students' reading of outstanding contributions to feminist work on health by those who adopt a largely qualitative approach (Oakley 1974, 1979, 1981; Bart 1981; Graham 1986, 1987c). How could anyone wanting to know about women's feelings on episiotomy, for instance, prefer a five-point scale from 'loved it' to 'hated it' to the sensitive interpretations made by Ann Oakley of the responses given to her in her study of the transition to early motherhood? But to compare the best of qualitative research with the crudest of quantitative research avoids important issues about the generation, use, and analysis of large-scale data. As Audrey Hunt has pointed out, 'We do not help social research into questions affecting women . . . by calling each other head shrinkers and number crunchers' (Hunt 1986: 19). Ann Oakley describes in her chapter some of the problems of this quantitative/qualitative divide, making the important point that if quantitative research is to be out of bounds for those professing a feminist approach, the result is a restriction on the sorts of questions which may be asked. 'This restriction may very well be counter to the same epistemological goal a code of feminist research practice is designed to promote' (Chapter 7).

THE DEMOCRATIC STATISTIC

The anti-authoritarian nature of statistics can take at least two forms. Statistics can expose the deficiencies of existing orthodoxies – they can, in other words, be part of the reasoned conduct of enquiry based on evidence. But in that sense they challenge not authority, but simply the authority of an existing view. Conducted amongst experts, such controversies do not challenge the authority of those who pronounce on matters of public policy, since they are themselves a part of its authoritative development. But there is another kind of challenge. This is when it is recognized that the authority of science lies in its evidence and its arguments. Once it is recognized that information is potentially available and understandable for the ordinary citizen, then science has truly become anti-authoritarian. It becomes part of the citizen's denial of a blank cheque to those in public positions to write whatever interpretation of information they choose.

A good example of the way in which data supplied by specialists can be put to use by non-professionals is given in Alison Macfarlane's chapter where she describes the decline in the number of labours induced through the use of oxytocin. The publication of research which failed to show a benefit in the use of oxytocin was used to good effect by groups campaigning against what they felt was an excess of induction, and the rate of induction fell.

The use of statistics can thus be part of either de-skilling or empowerment, a closure of the world of public enquiry, or a further instrument in the hands of the active and intelligent citizen. This is so whichever of the current models – of politics and citizenship, or markets and consumers – one uses for the understanding of health provision and promotion. If women are citizens, then they need the fullest information, not simply dispensed authoritatively, but available for selection, interpretation, and critical use, in order fully to act in that role. If they are consumers – and they are perhaps the largest class of health consumers who are at the same time health providers, and hence consumers in their own right and on behalf of others – then to work efficiently, markets need the fullest possible information. To that extent, the broad choices between politics and markets do not affect the need for both the availability of statistical information and a critical understanding of the way that it is, or could be used.

The combination of an awareness of the specific dimension of gender together with the greater salience of public decisions on health has created a sharper definition of women's health, not just in terms of private lifestyles, but as a specific issue in public policy. It is perhaps ironic that this process has been assisted by the politicization of health which has been one result of government proposals over the last ten years. The move to take issues of social policy out of politics and into the market has led to a renewed and vigorous discussion of the public dimension of both the causes and treatment of ill health, and the promotion and conditions of good health. This collection of essays will, I hope, contribute to that discussion.

Chapter Two

OFFICIAL STATISTICS AND WOMEN'S HEALTH AND ILLNESS[1]

ALISON MACFARLANE [2]

This exploration of what official 'health statistics' can tell us about women focuses mainly on statistics for England and Wales. Although Scotland has a more comprehensive system of official statistics, the context in which they are collected has much in common with that south of the border.

The phrase 'health statistics' is inevitably a loose one. Despite attempts made by the World Health Organisation and others, there is no commonly agreed definition of 'health'. This makes it unrealistic to expect statistics to measure it. It would probably be more appropriate to describe the data as 'medical statistics' or, increasingly, 'health service statistics'. Also, as we shall see, they tell us more about death and the use of health services than they do about health or ill health.

The actual and potential ability of official statistics to give us information about women's ill health cannot be assessed without an understanding of the process by which the data come to be collected and analysed. The Government Statistical Service reflects the way that, in its own words, it 'exists to serve the needs of government'. This priority, which was strengthened in 1981 in the aftermath of Sir Derek Rayner's review of the Government Statistical Service, has a long history. Despite attempts made in the nineteenth century to collect information about health through the census and other routine sources, the first conscious attempt to make an official study of the health of the population was prompted by the unfitness of potential recruits for the Boer War (Interdepartmental Committee on Physical Deterioration 1904).

Because of the way that they are increasingly shaped by the demands of the government, official statistics are anything but neutral, objective, and value-free. In any case, the way most official statistics are collected, as by-products of administrative and legal processes, can limit the extent to which they can be used for purposes other than those originally envisaged (Miles and Irvine 1979).

The way these constraints can affect medical statistics has been recognized for many years. William Farr, who set up the system for analysing birth and death registration statistics for England and Wales, put it this way in 1839, in the first annual report of the Registrar General:

> The registration of births and deaths proves the connexion of families, facilitates the legal distribution of property, and answers several other public purposes, which sufficiently establish its utility but in the performance of the duty with which you have been pleased to entrust me, I have to examine the registration under a different point of view, and with different objects, which will ultimately prove of not less importance. The deaths, and causes of death, are scientific facts which admit of numerical analysis; and science has nothing to offer more inviting in speculation than the laws of vitality, the variations of those laws in the two sexes at different ages, and the influence of civilisation, occupation, locality, seasons and other physical agencies, either in generating diseases and inducing death, or in improving the public health.
>
> (Farr 1839)

As Willam Farr predicted, official statistics have been invaluable on countless occasions over the past 150 years and will continue to be so, despite their limitations. This chapter starts by looking at these in more detail before going on to look at what they can tell us about the relation between women's health and our paid employment. It then discusses what they can tell us about women's health in general and ends by looking at comparisons between women and men.

THE NATURE OF OFFICIAL STATISTICS

Because of the way official statistics are collected through government and the National Health Service, they mainly record information about people to whom some event has happened, such as illness, injury, death, or birth. The routes through which this information is collected are summarized in Figure 2.1. Further information can be found in the Central Statistical Office's *Guide to Official Statistics* (1986) and Radical Statistics Health Group's *The Unofficial Guide to Official Health Statistics* (1981). Much more detailed accounts can be found in the relevant volumes of *Reviews of UK Statistical Sources* (Selman 1988; Benjamin 1989) and in *Birth Counts: Statistics of Pregnancy and Childbirth* (Macfarlane and Mugford 1984).

Women are under-represented in official statistics generally (Oakley and Oakley 1979; Nissel 1980) and this is reflected in statistics about health and health care. An example of this is the way that, for many years, the numbers of claims for sickness absence benefits were used as a measure of trends in morbidity. These data cover only people entitled to claim full benefit, and thus exclude people who are not in paid employment, or who work part time and do not pay the full National Insurance contribution. With successive changes in the system which have led to an increasing use of self-certification for short-term illnesses, these data come to present such an incomplete picture that they can no longer be used to monitor trends.

Figure 2.1 also mentions surveys of the population at large. Many government surveys may not differ greatly in their nature from those done outside government. It has been suggested that surveys initiated by government can be more subject to sexism in the choice of topic, questions, and data analysis than those done by, say, academic departments but this may reflect an over-optimistic view of academic departments. Given the extent to which the latter are funded by government departments and research councils, this distinction is increasingly unlikely.

Certainly the upper echelons of the Civil Service as a whole and the Government Statistical Service in particular are very male dominated, even though the Office of Population Censuses and Surveys has had a woman as Registrar General and, over the past twenty years, has always had women in senior positions particularly in its Social Survey division. As Table 2.1 shows, men also predominate in the senior levels of the medical profession, despite increasing proportions of women. This is particularly true in the more powerful and glamorous specialities, such as surgery,

Figure 2.1 Types of official statistics

Source of Data	Examples	Characteristics
Civil registration	Births, stillbirths, marriages, deaths	Comprehensive coverage as documents required for legal purposes. Inflexible as questions can only be changed by Act of Parliament.
Statutory notifications	Births, infectious diseases	Coverage should be complete as notification required by law, but underreporting does occur especially with infectious diseases which cannot be notified unless the person consults a doctor.
Voluntary notifications	Cancer registration, congenital malformations	More underreporting but more opportunity to collect data than with statutory notifications and registrations.
Claims for National Insurance & Social Security benefits	Sickness absence, industrial injury, and accidents	Sickness absence statistics confined to those paying full National Insurance contributions. Industrial illness and accident benefits can only be paid if it can be readily established that the condition was occupational in origin – this is difficult for some occupational diseases.
Administrative returns to central government health departments	Waiting list returns	Emphasis on use and availability of service and facilities rather than on characteristics of those who use them.
Patients' contacts with the health service	Hospital Episode System, National Morbidity Survey	Data concentrate on hospital in-patients with fewer data about out-patients and very unrepresentative data from general practice. Because of the incompleteness of record linkage, data tend to deal with facilities and treatment rather than outcome.
Special analyses and record linkage	Registrar General's Decennial Supplement, OPCS Longitudinal Study	Combined analyses of data from more than one source, e.g. death registration and census. Much more powerful than data from single source but problems may arise when discrepancies arise in data e.g. different occupation given at census and death registration. The OPCS Longitudinal Study overcomes this but has much smaller numbers in its 1 per cent sample
Surveys (a) 'one-off' (b) continuous	Breast feeding, dental health General Household Survey	Includes people who have not been in contact with the health services. Continuous surveys enable trends to be monitored over time. The General Household Survey is the only continuously operated government data collection system which deals with people's own perceptions of their ill health.

medicine, and obstetrics, whose views of health and illness strongly affect the medical questions which are included in data collection systems, despite the increasing role of managers in the National Health Service. In any case, men greatly outnumber women in senior positions in NHS management (Equal Opportunities Review 1987; Homans 1989). On the other hand, women and people from ethnic minorities tend to have the lowest paid and least prestigious jobs (Harding 1989; Radical Statistics Health Group 1987). Having said this, it cannot be assumed that having women in top positions will be of benefit to other women, nor, given the growth of formal equal opportunities strategies, that white men will inevitably act to put women and people from ethnic minorities at a disadvantage.

A possible further source of under-reporting in official statistics and surveys is that knowing that information is being collected for the government may inhibit the way people respond. Despite this, people seem willing to answer questions on personal matters in government social surveys. In any case, problems are particularly likely to arise when collecting information about illegal practices, such as the use of certain drugs or sensitive subjects such as domestic violence.

Taking this as an example, people, mainly but not exclusively women, who are injured as a result of domestic violence are likely to be under-represented in official statistics, because of reluctance to disclose how their injuries arose. For the same reason, their numbers will be under-represented in the numbers of assaults reported to the police, the numbers of court actions brought and the numbers of applications for rehousing on the grounds of domestic violence. This is because these statistics only include the people who are aware of the possibilities, wish to take the action, and are able to obtain assistance from the relevant agencies. Similar points can be made about most other statistics about the use of statutory services and agencies. Further gaps are arising from the increasing role of voluntary and private agencies, most of whom have never kept statistics in any systematic way about people who use their services, or published the statistics they have kept. It is important both to encourage them to keep their own statistics and for government to extend its own data collection systems to include them.

Table 2.1 Percentage of women among selected grades of full- and part-time doctors and nurses, England, 1977 and 1986

Grade	Percentage who were women	
	1977	*1986*
Doctors:		
Hospital doctors	18.0	24.8
Consultant and senior hospital medical officer with allowance	9.6	13.6
Senior registrar	18.9	24.9
Registrar	17.8	23.1
Senior house officer	22.9	33.6
House officer	30.6	42.6
General practitioners:	15.6	15.0
Unrestricted principals	14.1	13.5
Trainees and others	36.7	35.4
Community health:	53.8	57.1
Community medicine	29.8	36.0
Clinical grades	57.9	72.3
Hospital nurses and midwives (numbers):	89.9	89.9
Registered nurses	83.3	84.7
Student nurses	88.2	89.7
Enrolled nurses	90.8	91.9
Pupil nurses	92.2	93.4
Other nurses	95.1	92.8
Midwives	100.0	100.0
Whole-time	84.9	85.2
Part-time	98.2	98.6

Source: Health and Personal Social Services Statistics for England (DHSS 1978; Department of Health 1988)

Note: These data come from the Department of Health's main annual volume of statistics. It does not tabulate other types of NHS staff by sex. Other data sources which do so show that women and black people are more likely to be found in the lowest paid jobs (Equal Opportunities Review, 1987).

Even conditions which lead to consultations with NHS medical staff can be underreported, particularly if there is a stigma attached and if they are not necessarily easy to diagnose. This is certainly true of AIDS, where people may die of the condition without being diagnosed, or people with HIV infection may die of conditions not yet recognized as being associated with the virus. In England and Wales, in recent years, there have been increases in death-rates in single men in the 15–54 age group, but not in women. Although not certified as being due to AIDS, it is strongly suspected that the excess deaths are a consequence of it, and that the difference between the sexes probably arises from the much lower incidence of HIV infection among women in England and Wales (McCormick 1988).

In government, the nature of statistics can be affected by the way their compilation is organized. Staff working either on different stages in producing the same statistics, or producing complementary statistics on related subjects, can sometimes find themselves isolated from each other, either if they are separated geographically, or if the work is organized in a compartmentalized way (Government Statisticians' Collective 1979).

Except where surveys are done, the ways official statistics are collected make them unsuited to dealing with questions which are qualitative rather than quantitative. Thus, for example, routine data collection systems can be designed to count the numbers of people who had a particular treatment or operation, but they are not a very good way of trying to find out people's views of their treatment. Equally, they cannot tell us whether one treatment is better than another. This is more appropriately investigated through randomized trials, while other questions can be approached through case control studies, prospective studies of defined populations, and other epidemiological techniques. Apart from surveys, the most important role of official statistics is to monitor trends and variations in factors associated with ill health and in the care which is provided. The process of doing this can often highlight questions which need to be tackled by other means.

PROBLEMS IN RECORDING AND CLASSIFYING WOMEN'S OCCUPATIONS

Although progress has been made since 1980 when this review of official statistics and women's health was first written for the Equal Opportunities Commission (Macfarlane 1980), one of the biggest gaps in the information about women in official statistics is about the association between their paid employment and their health. This is because of the tendency not to collect information about women's occupations. The *Registrar General's Decennial Supplement on Occupational Mortality in the years 1979–80 and 1982–83* quotes instructions to registrars in England and Wales about death registration:

In the case of married and widowed women both the woman's own occupation and the occupation of her husband should be recorded. For all other women only their own occupation should be recorded. However registrars are advised that the occupation of a woman should not be recorded unless she was in paid employment most of her life.
(Office of Population Censuses and Surveys 1986a)

Interestingly, as it pointed out, this does not apply in Scotland where 'no distinction is made between males and females in the collection of information on employment' (Office of Population Censuses and Surveys 1986a). For children under 16 dying in England and Wales, both parents' occupations are now recorded at death registration, but before 1982 only fathers' occupations were recorded. Mothers' occupations were not recorded at birth registration before 1986, unless they were registering a birth outside marriage without the baby's father. Since then, mothers should have been asked if they want their occupation recorded at birth registration. In a considerable proportion of instances, this information is missing, although the position is improving. At the time of writing, new legislation is being planned which will provide an explicit place on birth certificates for mothers' occupations (Office of Population Censuses and Surveys 1988a). If these proposals are enacted, they may well increase the completeness of reporting.

Many data collection systems, including the Hospital Episode System and its predecessor the Hospital In-patient Enquiry, do not collect any information about the socio-economic status of the people they cover. The General Household Survey records occupations of all economically active women, but all published tabulations in the health section relate married women living in the same household as their husbands to socio-economic groups derived from their husbands' occupations.

This practice has been much criticized, and sometimes in exaggeratedly simple terms such as:

To the government statistician, the most important thing about a married woman is still her husband's occupation, not her own. The latest General Household Survey shows the farcical results that this demeaning view of women produces.
(unsigned article in *New Society* 1978)

25

The problem is more serious than this implies, however. The shortage of data makes it difficult either to monitor women's occupational health hazards (McDowall 1983, 1985) or assess whether their health problems are associated with the way their own or their husbands' occupations measure their socio-economic circumstances. The solutions are by no means as simple as the quotation above would seem to imply.

These problems have been with us for some time. John Tatham, one of William Farr's successors, wrote in the *Registrar General's Decennial Supplement for 1901*:

> Now that the industrial employment of women elsewhere than in the home has come to be so largely regulated by the state there is a manifest need for definite information respecting the occupational mortality of women workers. . . In the interval elapsed since the publication of the previous supplement so great has been the advance of public interest concerning the female occupation, especially in relation to the closely allied question of excessive mortality among infants, that in making preparation for the present supplement it was decided to submit the question of female occupational mortality to a test more exhaustive than any that had been previously applied.
>
> (Tatham 1908)

Unfortunately, he found that although occupations were recorded for 34.5 per cent of women aged over 15 enumerated in the 1901 census, only 8.0 per cent of those who died in the years 1900, 1901, or 1902 had occupations stated on their death certificate, making analyses problematic. The position was fairly similar seventy years later. In the 1971 census 42.2 per cent of married women aged 15–74 gave occupations, but occupations were stated for only 7.8 per cent of those who died in the years 1970–2. (Office of Population Censuses and Surveys 1978a). Ten years later reporting was much fuller, but still inadequate for analysis. According to the 1981 census, 60 per cent of women aged 20–59 and 26 per cent of those aged 60–74 were in paid employment. Of those who died in the years 1979–80 or 1982–83, 32 per cent of women aged 20–59 and 23 per cent of those aged 60–74 had occupations recorded at death registration (Office of Population Censuses and Surveys 1986a).

T. H. C. Stevenson, John Tatham's successor, was able to take advantage of new developments in information technology, in the form of the Hollerith counter sorter, to plan an extended range of analyses of the 1911 census. In describing these to a meeting of the Royal Statistical Society, he mentioned that married women's occupations would be included on the punched cards (Stevenson 1910). The data were used in analyses of infant mortality and fertility rather than the women's own occupational mortality (General Register Office 1923).

In the decennial supplement to the 1921 census, he proposed the idea of analysing married women's mortality according to their husbands' occupations. His main aim in doing this, however, was to interpret the statistics about men's mortality:

It will be found from the following pages that the effect of occupation upon male mortality is on the whole more direct than indirect – that mortality is influenced more by the conditions of life implied by various occupations than by the direct occupational risks entailed . . . It would therefore be possible to tabulate the mortality of 6–7 million married women by the occupation of their husbands. If this were done, we should for the first time, obtain a measure of the indirect effect (which in the case of females at all events, is almost entirely of chief importance) of occupation on mortality. This would not only be of importance for females, but would provide a means of roughly differentiating between the two different types of occupational influence upon males.

(Stevenson 1927)

These plans were put into effect in analysing the decennial supplement to the 1931 census when only 10 per cent of married women were 'recorded as gainfully employed' (General Register Office 1938). The decennial supplement to the 1971 census, when 42.2 per cent of married women had stated occupations, was the first to analyse married women's mortality according to their own occupations. It also discussed the fallacies of Stevenson's arguments about work and way of life. Not only can married women be harmed by the direct effects of their own occupations, but couples can affect each other directly by coming home from work with harmful substances on their clothes or skin. There are also other problems in trying to differentiate between the effects of work and 'way of life' (Office of Population Censuses and Surveys 1978a).

Compared with death certificates, two other official data collection systems have much fuller data about women's occupations. In its Longitudinal Study, the Office of Population Censuses and Surveys (OPCS) links death certificates with data collected at the previous census for a 1 per cent sample of the population of England and Wales. The General Household Survey, a continuous sample survey of the population of Great Britain, asks, among many other things, about people's current occupations and health problems. In both these cases, the sample is too small to gather information about mortality and morbidity in specific occupational groups. They are, however, used for the second purpose mentioned earlier, that of relating people's ill health to their socio-economic position as measured by classifications based on groups of occupations.

The first of these classifications was devised by T. H. C. Stevenson for use in analysing data from the 1911 census. In describing to the Royal Statistical Society how the classification had been modified for use in the 1921 census, he justified basing it on occupation rather than measures of wealth by citing the low mortality of clergymen. In his view, this 'seems to make it clear that the lower mortality of the wealthier classes depends less on wealth itself than upon the culture, extending to matters of hygiene, generally associated with it' (Stevenson 1928).

In the discussion which followed, a leading statistician of the time, Major Greenwood, commented that

> I think Dr Stevenson means by 'wealth' the purchasing power of the family unit, and by 'culture', not an acquaintance with differential equations or the minor poems of Horace, but a combination of knowledge and skill which enables a person to use his purchasing power wisely. . . . In any community such as ours there does exist a group of persons whose purchasing power is so small that no amount of 'culture' in Dr Stevenson's sense could possibly enable them to provide adequately for the family unit.
>
> (Greenwood 1928)

Although the Registrar General's social classes were put forward as a measure of 'culture' or 'way of life', the different but not unrelated concept of 'occupational status' was used to define them. They produced differences in mortality which Stevenson considered to be 'an indication both of success in the social grading of the population and of the association of mortality with low status' (Stevenson 1928). Although occupational classifications have been revised at successive censuses, the same principle, based on status, rather than wealth or relationship to the means of production has been applied on each occasion and social class differences in the mortality of men have persisted (Nichols 1979).

For women, the story is more complex. Many married women have occupations which are assigned to a different social class from those of their husbands and in some cases the woman is the main wage earner. As can be seen in Table 2.2, under half of the married women in paid employment enumerated in the 1981 census were assigned to the same class as their husband. Despite this, social class differences in mortality are still apparent when married women are tabulated according to their husbands' occupations, but little difference is seen when they are tabulated according to their own (McDowall 1983; Office of Population Censuses and Surveys 1986a). Similarly, differences can be seen in the measures of morbidity collected in the General Household Survey when married women are tabulated according to their husbands' socio-economic groups.

What does this mean? It could be concluded that married women's own socio-economic characteristics are less important than those of the husbands, but there are other factors which should be considered.

First, the social class classification was originally designed to produce a mortality gradient for the range of occupations done by men, and is probably inappropriate for classifying the very different range of occupations done by women (McDowall 1983). Much work has been done in the last few years to develop more appropriate ways of classifying women's occupations (Roberts and Barker 1987; Barker and Roberts 1986). In particular, within government, a new classification was developed by Jean Martin and Ceridwen Roberts (1984) in connection with their major survey of women and employment.

A second approach is to look for other socio-economic indicators which could be associated with women's ill health. Once

Table 2.2 Comparison of social classes of wives and husbands[1] living in private households, England and Wales 1981 (10% sample of 1981 census)

Social class of wife	Percentage of husbands in social class						Total[2]	Number in 10% sample	Percentage of wives in each class
	I	II	IIIn	IIIm	IV	V			
I Professional	51.4	30.3	7.8	7.4	2.5	0.6	100.0	4,538	0.9
II Intermediate	10.8	47.9	11.0	20.8	7.9	1.6	100.0	107,795	21.2
IIIn Skilled non-manual	6.5	27.7	16.2	34.8	12.2	2.7	100.0	196,344	38.6
IIIm Skilled manual	2.6	14.0	9.0	49.0	19.8	5.7	100.0	39,833	7.8
IV Partly skilled	2.3	13.1	8.1	46.6	23.2	6.7	100.0	117,038	23.0
V Unskilled	1.2	7.8	6.2	48.4	25.7	10.5	100.0	43,471	8.5
All classes	6.1	25.9	11.7	36.6	15.5	4.3	100.0	509,019	100.0

Source: OPCS Census 1981. Household and family composition. CEN 81 HFC Table 26A, 1984b

Note: [1] Excludes husbands and wives who were economically inactive, members of the armed forces, or whose occupations were inadequately described.
[2] Because of rounding, percentages may not add up to exactly 100.0

again, this activity has developed considerably over the past ten years. As far as data from official sources are concerned, much work has been done using the OPCS Longitudinal Study to look at factors associated with women's mortality. These show that other socio-economic indices, notably housing tenure and car ownership, need to be used in conjunction with data about women's own occupations and those of their husbands (Moser *et al.* 1988a). The General Household Survey has been used to look at the way women's health is associated with work in the home and paid work outside (Arber *et al.* 1985). These approaches are described in later chapters.

It is worth pointing out here that socio-economic indicators used in other countries may not be available in or appropriate to the United Kingdom. Data about the income of individuals or households are not readily available in a form which can be used in analyses of medical statistics. Years of education is commonly used as an indicator, but is a poor discriminator here where, up until recently, a very low proportion of the population has remained in full-time education beyond the statutory school leaving age.

Meanwhile, even if married women's occupations may not be a very powerful indicator of socio-economic status or correlate very closely with mortality or ill health, information about them is still needed to monitor specific occupational hazards. These can relate either to women's own mortality or to statistics about reproduction and babies, such as fertility, sex ratio, birthweight, congenital malformations, and perinatal and infant mortality (McDowall 1985).

STATISTICS SPECIFIC TO WOMEN

What, despite their drawbacks, do official statistics tell us about problems specific to women? Pregnancy is so often treated as an illness, that it is sometimes difficult to remember that it is not one. For most women, however, it is the first time in their lives that they come into intensive contact with the health services.

Despite the fact that the risk of having a stillbirth or losing a baby in the first year of life declined rapidly in the latter half of the 1970s and early 1980s, our perinatal and infant mortality rates have received a disproportionate amount of adverse publicity and are invariably misreported (Macfarlane and Mugford 1984; Macfarlane 1988a). Although the likelihood of having a successful outcome of pregnancy is closely associated with a woman's health and socio-economic circumstances, pregnancy may in its turn affect a woman's health.

The risk of dying from the consequences of pregnancy or childbirth is now very small, but up to just over fifty years ago, the position was very different, as Figure 2.2 shows. The picture is made more complicated by the changes in the definition of maternal mortality at successive revisions of the International Classification of Diseases. It also shows the increase in reporting in 1881 when the General Register Office introduced its system of 'medical enquiries'. Whenever it received a death registration relating to women of childbearing age, a letter was sent to the doctor who signed the certificate asking explicitly whether her death had been caused by pregnancy or childbirth.

From the mid-1930s onwards, the maternal mortality rate declined rapidly. In 1988, there were only 41 such deaths in England and Wales, a rate of only 5.9 per 100,000 maternities or 4.8 per 100,000 total maternities plus abortions. Maternal deaths are subjected to detailed investigation through the process of 'confidential enquiries'. The current system dates back to 1952, but has its origins in the 1920s and early 1930s. This was a time when maternal mortality was rising and was therefore a great matter of public concern, particularly among middle-class women who, unusually, had a greater risk of death than working-class women (General Register Office 1938).

Although contraception has undoubtedly played a part in the decline in maternal mortality, it too has its hazards. Valerie Beral (1979) reviewed these hazards and concluded that maternal mortality was no longer an adequate measure of deaths associated with reproduction. She proposed an alternative measure, the 'reproductive mortality rate', which included deaths from complications of contraceptive use as well as those from complications of pregnancy and abortion. Deaths from complications of pregnancy and childbirth fell between 1950 and 1975, as did deaths from abortion, particularly after the 1967 Abortion Act. For women aged 25–34 this more than offset the increase in mortality which could be attributed to oral contraceptives and, to a lesser extent, IUDs and sterilization. In the 35–44 age group,

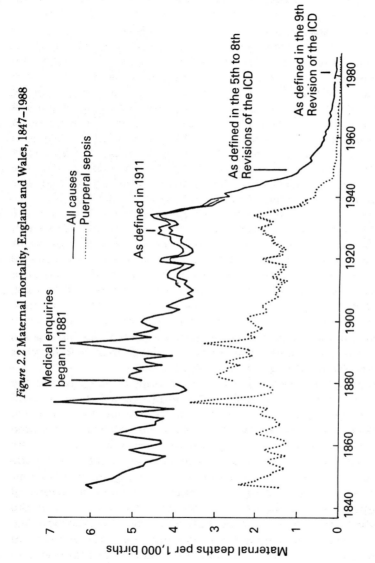

Figure 2.2 Maternal mortality, England and Wales, 1847–1988

Source: OPCS Mortality Statistics

however, mortality attributed to these methods of birth control increased markedly from 1960 onwards, and was greater than the fall in maternal mortality, and so the reproductive mortality rate rose.

These estimates of reproductive mortality could not be derived exclusively from routinely collected statistics, and the methods used point to a lack of data in some of these areas.

There are no sufficiently detailed routinely collected data about the use of different forms of birth control. Although the declining numbers of 'family planning' clinics collect data about the different methods used by their clients, less detailed information is collected about services provided by general practitioners because it is related to the 'item of service' payments made to GPs for providing contraceptive services. Thus only the insertion of IUDs is shown separately as this work commands a higher fee than consultations for all other types of contraception. The data from general practice are not analysed according to the women's ages, as this does not affect the fee paid. Sterilizations and vasectomies done under the NHS appear in the relevant hospital and clinic statistics, but no information is collected on a routine basis about those done in the private sector. This is an important omission, as two surveys done in 1981 and 1986 showed that these accounted for a sizeable, though declining number of sterilizations (Nicholl *et al* 1989a).

Valerie Beral based her estimates on two OPCS surveys done in 1970 and 1975 about the use of birth control services (Bone 1973, 1978), but even these were restricted to married women. This was fortunately not the case with OPCS' Family Formation Survey, done in 1976 (Dunnell 1979). Some questions from this survey were included in the 1983 and 1986 General Household Survey (Office of Population Censuses and Surveys 1985b, 1989a) which asked them of all women aged 16–49.

Data about legal abortion are rather more plentiful. Under the 1967 Abortion Act, all terminations of pregnancy should be notified to the Chief Medical Officers of England, Wales, or Scotland. Extensive analyses done by OPCS tell us, for example, that a quarter of the women living in England and Wales whose pregnancies were terminated in 1988 had two or more live born children, 99.4 per cent were terminated before the twenty-third week of pregnancy, 40.9 per cent of terminations were done under the NHS, and a further 5.7 per cent were done on non-NHS premises, at NHS expense, on an agency basis (Office of Population Censuses and Surveys 1989b).

On the other hand, these analyses cannot tell us how many of the remaining 53.4 per cent of women would have preferred an NHS abortion, had it been available, or why there have been more deaths among women having abortions under the NHS than in the private sector. This could reflect either differences in the quality of care or differences between the incidence of pre-existing medical complications in the two groups of women. This was a controversial issue ten years ago, but in the 1980s, the numbers of deaths have fallen so low in both sectors that comparisons are difficult to interpret and attract less attention.

Since the concept of reproductive mortality was first put forward, there have been changes in the nature and composition of oral contraceptives and a considerable body of further research has been done into their long-term side-effects. In some cases, the results are conflicting, as in the case of the possible association between oral contraceptives and breast cancer (Drife 1989). Also, new factors have entered the equation, and these would have to be taken into account in updating the estimates. Perhaps the most outstanding of these is the increasing use of drugs to treat infertility, and the increasing development and use of techniques for assisted reproduction. The side-effects of the drugs have yet to be fully investigated (Klein and Rowland 1989). Although there have yet been no reports of deaths associated with assisted reproduction in the United Kingdom, two have been reported in Australia, where these techniques are used much more frequently (Wood 1988; Lumley 1989).

Reproductive mortality is difficult enough to measure, but it would be even harder to define a global measure of reproductive morbidity. Furthermore, data about such problems as the non-fatal side-effects of contraceptive pill use or anxiety about an unwanted pregnancy are difficult to collect routinely, although much information has been obtained through *ad hoc* studies.

The increasingly technological nature of modern obstetrics and the concentration of births into large hospitals means that women are becoming more likely to be subjected to intervention in the course of pregnancy and delivery. It has to be remembered that there are circumstances in which the use of one or more of these procedures may make all the difference between whether or not a woman has a live healthy baby, others where there is no evidence to suggest that they make any difference whatsoever, and yet others where the practices may be positively harmful (Chalmers *et al.* 1989). Irrespective of the outcome for the baby, many procedures still have side-effects for the mother herself. For example women who have caesareans can develop post-operative infection and, if the operation resulted in a live birth, have to face the task of looking after a new baby after a major abdominal operation.

Unlike other countries, the caesarean rate in England and Wales levelled off at just above 10 per cent in the early 1980s, as Figure 2.3 shows. The reasons for this levelling off in the rising trend are unclear (Macfarlane 1988b). At the time of writing, rates for England for the years since 1985 have yet to emerge from the new maternity Hospital Episode System, which was set up on the recommendations of the Steering Group on Health Services Information (1985) to collect data about all in-patient stays in maternity hospitals in England.

Induction of labour by artificial rupture of the membranes, or use of oxytocin, or both, became increasingly used in the early 1970s, reaching a peak of 38.9 per cent of all women delivering in NHS hospitals in England and Wales in 1974 (Department of Health and Social Security, Office of Population Censuses and Surveys and Welsh Office 1980). After that the rate declined until in 1985 only 17.5 per cent of women delivering in NHS hospitals in England had labour induced (Department of Health and Social Security and Office of Population Censuses and Surveys 1988). When the induction rate first started to decline, it was difficult to monitor as the practice of using oxytocin and artificial rupture of membranes to augment, or speed up, labours which had started spontaneously was growing and some of the women concerned were wrongly coded as having had labour induced (Macfarlane and Mugford 1984). The reasons for the decline are probably the combination of the publication of research which failed to demonstrate any benefit in a policy of extensive use of induction (Chalmers *et al.* 1976) and found an association between oxytocin and jaundice in new-born babies (Chalmers *et al.* 1975), and the use of such research findings by groups campaigning against what they felt, with good reason, to be a too frequent use of induction.

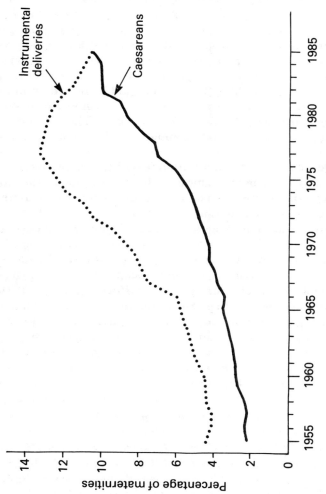

Figure 2.3 Trends in operative deliveries,
England and Wales 1955–85

Source: Maternity Hospital In-patient Enquiry, Welsh Office

There are other data, such as on the use of ultrasound investig-ations and amniocentesis tests during pregnancy, which are relevant but are not routinely collected on a national scale in England. Until recently there have been no consistent national data about the use of anaesthetics during labour. It is hoped that this will change once data start to emerge from the Hospital Episode System. What this will not do is tell us associations between events during labour and ill health after the mother has left hospital, such as postnatal depression, or pain resulting from either episiotomies or tears, and which can still be present several years later. It is unlikely that these would be picked up in routine statistics, unless they lead to admission to hospital in the NHS district in which the delivery took place. There is no routine linkage between information about care given in hospital and care given by GPs.

Despite their limitations, routine statistics about pregnancy and childbirth are more complete than those about the possible associations between women's activities at home in childrearing, giving 'informal' and usually unpaid care to sick or elderly relatives, and combining these with paid employment outside their homes. The *Women and Employment* survey (Martin and Roberts 1984) found that 13 per cent of women under 60 had respons-ibility for sick, disabled, or elderly people. Since then, analysis of General Household Survey data for 1985 (Green 1988) showed that women aged between 30 and 64 were more likely than men to be acting as carers for another adult, and more likely to be acting as the main carer, as Table 2.3 shows. Other research has found that male carers were more likely than women to receive outside help from statutory and voluntary services (Parker 1985). Over the past five years, a fuller picture of these activities has emerged from the General Household Survey and is discussed in chapter 3.

There is a complete dearth of official statistics about women's health problems during and following the menopause. Medical care for these is usually given by general practitioners or gynae-cology out-patient clinics. In both settings, relatively few statistics are collected routinely. These consultations can lead to surgery, and there is an increasing tendency for operations such as hyster-ectomy to take place in private hospitals (Nicholl *et al.* 1989a) where no statistics are collected routinely. This leaves a sizeable gap in the national information base, as, for example, a special survey estimated that just over a fifth of all hysterectomies done in 1986 in women living in England and Wales were in private hospitals (Nicholl *et al.* 1989b).

Table 2.3 Percentage of adults who were carers, Great Britain, 1985

Type of care. Percentage of adults who were:	Sex	Age, years 16–29	30–44	45–64	65 and over	Total
Caring for some-	Male	2	3	5	6	4
one in the same	Female	2	3	7	5	4
household*						
Caring for some-	Male	4	8	11	8	8
one in another	Female	5	13	17	8	11
private household only						
Main carers	Male	2	5	10	9	6
	Female	3	10	18	9	10
Caring for at least	Male	1	2	4	5	3
20 hours per	Female	1	4	6	4	4
week						
All carers	Male	6	11	16	14	12
	Female	7	16	24	12	15

Source: OPCS, General Household Survey, 1985 (Office of Population Censuses and Surveys 1987)

Note. * Includes people who were caring for someone in the same household and also someone in another private household.

Rather more data are available about cancer, through regional cancer registries and the National Cancer Registration Scheme, although the data are of variable quality, and changes in registration rates can be difficult to interpret. For example, in 1984 there was a marked increase in registration of cancer of the cervix (Office of Population Censuses and Surveys 1988b), but it is difficult to see to whether this relates to changes in registration practice, changes in incidence, or to screening activity.

Since then, new data collection systems have been introduced. As, at time of writing, data have yet to emerge from them, it is too soon to pass judgement on them. Concern has been expressed about the new system however. It may well be designed more to monitor activity than to provide epidemiological data which would enable the effectiveness of the programme to be assessed (Draper 1985). Given the concern about the variable quality of local screening services, there is clearly a need to monitor and assess what is happening (Day 1989; Smith *et al* 1989). Unfortunately, the abolition of the Committee on Gynaecological Cytology means that the prospects of this happening are not good (McPherson 1989).

DIFFERENCES BETWEEN MEN AND WOMEN

Tables 2.4 to 2.14 give a brief overview of what official statistics can tell us about differences between men and women. The limitations of the data sources described earlier should be borne in mind when trying to interpret them.

Table 2.4 Deaths per million population by age and sex, England and Wales, 1986

| | Rate | | Ratio |
Age, years	Male	Female	Male/Female
All ages	11,175	10,743	1.04
Under 1	5,496	3,871	1.40
1–4	442	398	1.11
5–14	220	171	1.29
15–24	768	311	2.47
25–34	872	470	1.86
35–44	1,674	1,121	1.49
45–54	5,267	3,227	1.63
55–64	16,603	9,245	1.79
65–74	42,891	23,443	1.83
75–84	101,069	62,530	1.62
85+	214,713	171,003	1.26

Source: OPCS Mortality Statistics, Series DH2, No. 13, 1988e

Women have a longer expectation of life than men. The expectation of life at birth in 1985 was 77.4 years for women in England and Wales, compared with 71.5 for men (Central Statistical Office 1989). In addition, as Table 2.4 shows, the overall mortality rate for women is lower than that for men in every age group. Table 2.5 shows that the percentages of men and women whose deaths were attributed to conditions in each of the main categories of causes of death were roughly similar in 1986. Compared with ten years earlier, there was a reduction in the percentage of deaths of men and women attributed to respiratory disease and accidents and violence, but an increase in those attributed to mental disorders. This reflects the increasing proportion of deaths attributed to senile dementia, particularly for women. It is a moot point as to whether these changes reflect changes in the prevalence of the conditions, or changes in views about appropriate ways to certify causes of death.

Within age groups, however, there are considerable differences in death rates, as Table 2.6 shows. For example, between the ages of 35 and 64, mortality attributed to diseases of the circulatory system is about three times higher for men than for women, but the difference narrows for the much higher rates of death in the older age groups (Office of Population Censuses and Surveys 1988e). One way of summarizing this is to look at it in terms of 'years of life lost': either 'years of working life lost', between the ages of 15 and 64, or 'years of total life lost', taking the age of 90 as an upper limit (Office of Population Censuses and Surveys 1989c). These are higher for men than women. Although 'years of working life lost' attributed to heart disease, motor vehicle accidents, and suicide are much higher for men than for women, the position of the two sexes is fairly similar for cancer.

The importance of looking within age groups and groups defined by other characteristics cannot be stressed too strongly, as looking only at overall rates can lead to incorrect interpretation, as in this example:

> . . . many women risk their health both physically and psychologically in the performance of domestic labour. Women at home have a high accident rate, and the undercapitalised and isolated nature of housework is an important contributory factor in this. In 1971, 6245 people died in home accidents – 35.3 per cent of whom were men and 64.7 per cent women – while many more were injured. Naturally none of these figures appear in the industrial accident statistics since domestic labour is not officially counted as work.

> (Doyal and Pennell 1979)

In 1986, the total numbers of people dying from accidents at home had fallen, but the difference between men and women persisted. The breakdown by age group, however, shows a

Table 2.5 Certified causes of death among men and women of all ages, England and Wales, 1976 and 1986

Cause group	1976			1986		
	ICD codes 8th revision	Percentage of deaths Men	Women	ICD codes 9th revision	Percentage of deaths Men	Women
Neoplasms (cancers)	140–239	22.7	19.7	140–239	25.6	22.9
Mental disorders	290–315	0.2	0.4	290–319	1.4	2.8
Diseases of the circulatory system	390–458	48.5	51.8	390–459	47.4	48.5
Diseases of the respiratory system	460–519	16.3	15.4	460–519	11.5	10.2
Accidents and violence	E800–999	3.9	3.1	E800–999	3.9	2.6
All other causes		8.4	9.6		10.2	13.0
Total		100.0	100.0		100.0	100.0
Number of deaths		300,058	298,458		287,894	293,309

Source: OPCS Mortality Statistics, cause. Series DH2, Nos 3 and 13, 1978c and 1988b

Table 2.6 Deaths per million population by age and sex, England and Wales 1986

Cause (ICD ninth revision)	Sex	All ages	Under 1 year	1–4	5–14	15–24	25–34	35–44	45–54	55–64	65–74	75–84	85+
All causes	M	11,175	5,496	442	220	768	872	1,674	5,267	16,603	43,891	101,069	214,713
	F	10,743	3,871	398	171	311	470	1,121	3,227	9,245	23,443	62,530	171,003
Neoplasms (140–239)	M	2,926	(32)	43	41	70	128	392	1,487	5,461	12,954	23,247	31,232
	F	2,560	(31)	51	43	50	170	592	1,806	4,199	7,418	11,546	17,286
Mental disorders (290–319)	M	154	(3)	(4)	(2)	17	24	21	21	57	340	2,121	6,648
	F	292	(3)	(2)	(2)	6	6	8	14	51	290	1,952	8,114
Diseases of the circulatory system (390–459)	M	5,332	62	(15)	(10)	31	106	553	2,593	8,277	21,443	50,009	101,986
	F	5,194	75	(15)	(8)	21	52	175	710	3,153	11,100	34,134	91,888
Diseases of the respiratory system (460–519)	M	1,255	633	30	8	22	31	62	207	1,100	4,272	19,380	45,135
	F	1,079	397	26	10	15	18	41	131	640	1,720	5,870	26,987
Accidents and violence (E800–999)	M	451	188	109	89	522	457	417	467	498	632	1,323	3,174
	F	280	157	86	52	142	132	143	209	256	435	1,068	3,018
All other causes	M	1,057	4,578	241	70	106	126	229	492	1,210	3,340	9,989	26,538
	F	1,338	3,208	218	56	77	92	162	357	946	2,480	7,960	23,710

Source: OPCS Mortality Statistics, cause, 1986. Series DH2, No.13, 1988e

Note: Figures in brackets are based on less than 20 cases

different picture. Women aged 15–74 are less likely than men to have fatal accidents at home, but they are more likely to do so at ages of 75 or over, as Table 2.7 shows (Office of Population Censuses and Surveys 1989d). Thus housework is hardly likely to be the sole cause. The 1984 General Household Survey showed that women aged 65 and over were more likely to have accidents at home, but there was no difference between the sexes under the age of 65 (Office of Population Censuses and Surveys (1986b). On the other hand, women at all ages are more likely to have accidents at home which lead to admission to hospital (Department of Health and Social Security, Office of Population Censuses and Surveys 1987b).

Table 2.7a Deaths from accidents in the home, England and Wales, 1986

Age	Men		Women	
	Number	*Rate per million*	*Number*	*Rate per million*
All	2081	85.3	2458	95.7
Under 1 year	32	95.2	28	87.8
1–4	69	53.2	55	44.6
5–14	34	10.6	20	6.6
15–44	584	52.4	305	28.0
45–64	454	68.2	312	76.3
65–74	278	141.2	322	129.3
75+	630	571.8	1414	645.2

Source: OPCS. Mortality Statistics : accidents and violence. Series DH4 No.12, 1988d

Table 2.7b Estimated numbers of hospital discharges and deaths after injuries caused by accidents at home, England, 1985

Age	Men		Women	
	Number	*Rate per 10,000*	*Number*	*Rate per 10,000*
All	31380	1.4	50160	2.1
0–4	9840	64.6	6700	46.2
5–14	3990	13.0	3180	10.9
15–44	7460	7.2	7520	7.4
45–64	3280	5.2	4720	12.1
65–74	2300	12.6	5910	25.5
75–84	3000	34.0	12570	79.1
85+	1510	111.8	9560	214.4

Sources: DHSS, OPCS, Hospital In-patient Enquiry. Main tables Series MB4 No.27, 1987b

Statistics about the use of health services give the impression that women make greater use of health services than men. Although admission rates to acute, or non-psychiatric, hospitals are higher among women than men overall, admission rates are higher for boys under 15 and men aged 45 and over. Although admissions to maternity wards are specifically excluded from Table 2.8, many other admissions in this age group are much more closely related to reproduction than to illness. When abortions, miscarriages, and diseases of the male and female genital organs are excluded, the differences between men and women in the 15–44 age group virtually disappear.

Women living in private households tend to consult GPs about health problems more often than men, although, as Table 2.9 shows, the most marked difference is once again in the child-bearing age range (Office of Population Censuses and Surveys 1989a). Table 2.10 shows a slightly different story. It is based on consultations with a set of volunteer GPs who took part in the National Morbidity Survey (Royal College of General Practitioners, Office of Population Censuses and Surveys and Department of Health and Social Security 1986). The differences were much smaller once consultations which were not for illnesses were removed, and virtually disappeared after consultations for pregnancy and childbirth and diseases of the male and female genito-urinary systems were excluded.

The reasons for the consultations were also classified as 'serious', 'intermediate', and 'trivial'. Whereas consultation rates for 'serious' complaints were higher for women than men overall, rates for boys under the age of 5 and men aged over 64 were higher than those for girls and women in the corresponding age groups. For complaints labelled as 'intermediate' and 'trivial', consultation rates were higher for women than men in every age group except the under-5s. It is ironic that as all the consultations for matters which were not illnesses were labelled as 'trivial', many of these were for birth control or antenatal care! It has been suggested that one reason why women may consult more often for minor complaints is that they are more likely to take children to the doctor. Once there, they may take the opportunity of asking advice about a matter that would not on its own have prompted a visit.

Table 2.8 Hospital in-patient discharge rates, England, 1985

| | Sex | All | Discharge rates per 10,000 population — Age, years | | | | | | |
			0–4	5–14	15–44	45–64	65–74	75–84	85+
All causes	M	1032.1	1757.3	717.3	559.0	1080.5	2119.7	3353.2	4860.8
	F	1114.5	1230.7	522.3	905.6	1014.1	1504.8	2457.7	3741.4
Diseases of breast and genital organs (600–629)	M	38.2	68.8	39.8	16.8	32.8	99.0	136.4	122.1
	F	115.6	2.4	3.0	169.7	154.1	66.4	47.8	27.6
Abortion, miscarriage and conditions arising from childbearing (630–676)	F	60.7	0.5	1.8	142.6	1.2	0.1	0.5	1.1
Remaining causes	M	993.9	1694.5	677.5	542.2	1047.7	2020.7	3216.8	4738.7
	F	938.2	1227.8	517.6	593.3	858.8	1438.3	2409.4	3712.7

Source: DHSS, OPCS. Hospital In-Patient Enquiry 1985. Summary tables Series MB4 No.26, 1987a

Table 2.9 Differences in the use of health services by sex and age, Great Britain, 1976 and 1986

| Age, years | Consulted GP in 14 days before interview | | | | Percentage who attended out-patients or casualty in a 3-month reference period | | | | An in-patient stay in hospital during a 12-month period | | | |
| | 1976 | | 1986 | | 1976 | | 1986 | | 1976 | | 1986 | |
	M	F	M	F	M	F	M	F	M	F	M	F
0–4	12	13	21	21	10	8	12	11			11	9
5–15*	7	6	10	10	8	6	11	11			7	6
16–44*	8	14	7	17	9	8	13	11	Question not		6	14
45–64	11	11	13	15	10	11	15	16	asked in 1976		8	8
65–74	12	14	17	17	11	11	16	18			12	10
75+	13	17	22	22	11	10	19	18			18	15
Total	9	12	11	16	9	9	13	13			8	11

Source: OPCS General Household Survey, 1986 (1989a)
Note: * These age groups were 5–14 and 15–44 in 1976

Table 2.10 People consulting general practitioners in selected practices in the year July 1981–June 1982

| Cause of consultation | Sex | All ages | Rates per 1,000 persons at risk | | | | | | | |
			0–4	5–14	15–24	25–44	45–64	65–74	75+
All causes	M	652.2	991.3	661.3	582.6	579.4	630.9	720.7	777.1
	F	765.8	977.5	676.4	819.4	766.9	716.7	753.0	795.0
All illnesses	M	629.3	943.3	644.6	561.1	554.3	610.5	703.7	755.0
	F	718.1	918.3	657.8	722.1	695.6	695.1	738.3	778.3
Diseases of the genito-urinary system (ICD 580–629)	M	28.7	45.8	22.4	18.2	21.2	28.1	50.5	74.9
	F	138.9	36.1	37.6	197.9	224.2	137.7	65.7	66.6
Conditions of pregnancy, childbirth and the puerperium (630–676)	F	15.7		0.3	41.2	33.4	0.6		
All other illnesses	M	600.6	897.5	622.2	542.9	533.3	582.4	653.2	680.1
	F	563.5	882.2	619.9	483.0	438.0	557.4	672.6	711.7

Source: Royal College of GPs, OPCS, and DHSS (1986). Morbidity statistics from general practice 1981–2. Third national study. Series MB5 No. 1, 1986

Despite women's higher consultation rates with GPs, it is interesting to see from Table 2.9 that there is little difference in attendance rates at out-patient clinics. Data collected in the 1978 General Household Survey (Office of Population Censuses and Surveys 1980) showed a much greater use of medication by women, and it appeared that the excess was in prescribed rather than unprescribed drugs. The 1986 General Household Survey showed that equal proportions of men and women who had visited the doctor were given prescriptions, suggesting the difference resulted from women's higher consultation rates. Differences in in-patient stays showed a broadly similar pattern to those in Table 2.8.

How do the data about the use of health services relate to statistics about women's health? Women living in private households interviewed in the General Household Survey are no more likely to report chronic ill health than men, as Table 2.17 shows. It is interesting, however, that when the questions were changed in 1977 and 1978 to take the form of a check-list, reported ill health became more common, particularly among women. Not surprisingly, OPCS found this difficult to interpret (Office of Population Censuses and Surveys 1979). It was suggested that some of the items on the check-list, which were fairly common chronic health problems, such as backache, would not have been categorized by informants as 'long-standing illness, disability and infirmity'. In 1979, the original questions were reinstated, and the level of reported ill health dropped again, though in the 1980s it is consistently higher than in the 1970s, among men and women of all ages, as Table 2.12 shows.

Routinely collected statistics tell us relatively little about the prevalence of disability in the population. Even where registers are kept of people with specific disabilities, they are very often incomplete (Hey 1980; Johnson and King 1990). To fill this gap, the Office of Population Censuses and Surveys is asked from time to time to do special surveys. A major study of disability, consisting of four separate surveys, was done between 1985 and 1988 (Martin *et al.* 1988; Bone and Meltzer 1989). These covered adults and children living in private households and 'communal establishments' in Great Britain. The key concept was 'disability', which was defined as 'any restriction (resulting from an impairment) of ability to perform an activity in the manner or within the range considered normal for a human being' (Martin *et al.* 1988). In

Table 2.11 Differences in self-reported sickness by sex and age, Great Britain 1976 and 1986

| Age, years | Long-standing illness | | | | Percentage who reported limiting long-standing illness | | | | Restricted activity in 14 days before interview | | | |
| | 1976 | | 1986 | | 1976 | | 1986 | | 1976 | | 1986 | |
	M	F	M	F	M	F	M	F	M	F	M	F
0–4	8	6	12	11	2	2	3	4	10	8	15	12
5–15*	13	9	20	15	6	5	9	6	9	8	13	11
16–44*	17	17	24	24	9	9	11	12	9	10	10	13
45–64	37	35	44	46	25	23	27	28	9	9	12	16
65–74	52	54	58	61	38	40	41	43	9	11	15	18
75+	63	68	67	70	48	53	52	56	10	11	17	21
Total	25	26	32	34	15	17	18	21	9	10	12	14

Source: OPCS General Household Survey, 1986 (1989a)
Note: * These age groups were 5–14 and 15–44 in 1976.

Table 2.12 Percentages of people in each age group reporting chronic health problems, Great Britain
The effects of questions on response*

Age Group	1976 Male	1976 Female	Age Group	1977 Male	1977 Female	Age Group	1986 Male	1986 Female
15–44	17	17	16–44	45	62	16–44	24	24
45–64	37	35	45–64	65	75	45–64	44	46
65–74	52	54	65–74	74	81	65–74	58	61
75+	63	68	75+	79	85	70+	67	70

Source: OPCS, General Household Survey 1976, 1977, 1986 (Office of Population Censuses and Surveys 1978b, 1979, 1989a)

Note: * The questions asked were:

1976 and 1986 Do you have any long-standing illness disability or infirmity?

1977 Would you look at this card and tick in the boxes on the left any health problems that you yourself find keep recurring or that you have all the time?
Do you have any (other) health problem not on the list that keeps recurring or that you have all or most of the time?

contrast to this, the previous survey, done in 1969, had covered adults with impairments, which are defined as 'any loss of psychological, physiological or anatomical structure or function', and physical handicaps, living in private households (Harris 1971). Because, as a result, it covered a lower proportion of the population than the recent surveys and used different criteria for inclusion, it is difficult to assess trends over time.

In analysing the recent survey, a 10-point scale of severity of disability was developed. The most severely disabled people were given a rating of 10, and the least severely disabled a rating of 1. Cumulative prevalence rates are shown in Figure 2.4 and a closer look is taken at rates in people under 40 in Figure 2.5. Not surprisingly, the prevalence of disability increased with age for both men and women, but the differences between men and women showed a changing pattern. Under the age of 20, disability was more common in boys than in girls. After this, it was more common in women than men. At the least severe end of the scale, however, the relationship was reversed between the ages of 55 and 69. This happened between the ages of 65 and 79 for the most severe disabilities and between the ages of 55 and 70 for the least severe disabilities. The authors commented that 'The different retirement ages of men and women seem likely to be significant, but exactly what causes this difference is not clear' (Martin *et al.* 1988). They also discuss how their estimates of the prevalence of disability relate to the much more rudimentary measures collected through the General Household Survey.

Dentistry is an area of health care about which many routine statistics are produced, but as these are generated from the 'item of service' payments made to dentists, they tell us about the work which dentists did rather than about the people in whose mouths it was done. Information about this can, however, be found in a series of surveys of dental health done by OPCS. These include both questions to the respondents and a dental examination.

The survey of adult dental health done in 1978 (Todd and Walker 1980; Todd *et al.* 1982) found that more women than men had lost all their teeth before the age of 30 and the proportions of people with no teeth were higher in Scotland and the North of England than in the South. Women also had fewer sound teeth (defined as having neither decay nor fillings) than did men. A further survey of adult dental health was done in 1988. Meanwhile,

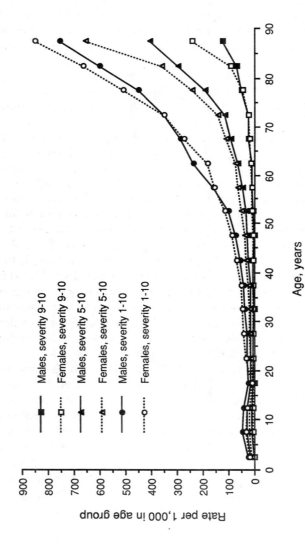

Figure 2.4 Disability by sex and severity, Great Britain 1985

Males, severity 9-10
Females, severity 9-10
Males, severity 5-10
Females, severity 5-10
Males, severity 1-10
Females, severity 1-10

Age, years

Rate per 1,000 in age group

Source: OPCS disability surveys

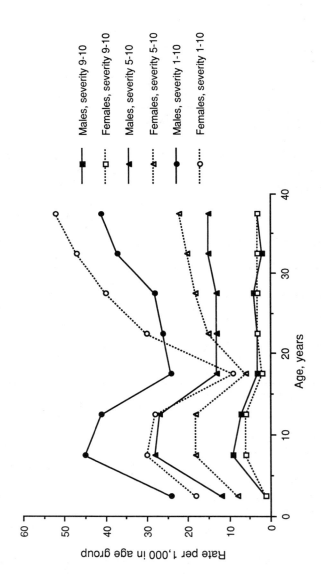

Figure 2.5 Disability by sex and severity up to the age of 40, Great Britain 1985

Males, severity 9-10
Females, severity 9-10
Males, severity 5-10
Females, severity 5-10
Males, severity 1-10
Females, severity 1-10

Rate per 1,000 in age group

Age, years

Source: OPCS disability surveys

questions on dental health were asked in the General Household Survey in 1983 and 1985. It was not, of course, possible to collect any detailed clinical information, but questions were asked about total tooth loss. Replies to these are compared with data from the 1968 and 1978 surveys in Table 2.13, which points to a continuing improvement in dental health, coupled with persisting differences between men and women (Office of Population Censuses and Surveys 1987), A higher proportion of women in each age group have no natural teeth, despite the fact that women who still have teeth left are more likely to visit dentists regularly.

The survey of children's dental health in 1983 did detailed analyses of geographical and class differences but did not look very closely at the differences between boys and girls. Perhaps not surprisingly, it found close associations betwen children's dental attendance patterns and those of their mothers (Todd and Dodd 1985).

Table 2.13 Percentage of each age and sex group who had no natural teeth

	England and Wales					
Age at interview	*1968*		*1978*		*1985*	
	Men	*Women*	*Men*	*Women*	*Men*	*Women*
25–34	6	8	3	4	1	2
35–44	16	28	9	14	5	6
45–54	36	44	24	33	15	19
55–64	61	66	41	56	34	44

Source: OPCS surveys of adult dental health, 1968–78 (Todd and Walker 1980).
General Household Survey 1985 (1987)

Any attempt at an assessment of the extent of mental ill health in a population is fraught with even greater problems than is measuring the extent of physical illness, as the judgements about the way the conditions are defined are even more subjective than with physical illness. There is often no clear agreement among doctors, nurses, and social workers. The problems are compounded when statistics are compiled, as they are based on a sum total of these value judgements.

The bulk of routine statistics are based on admissions to hospitals, although the new sets of statistics arising from the recommendations of the Steering Group on Health Services Information will include some new data about services provided in the community. Although hospital statistics include diagnoses, they do not tell us about the severity of the condition, nor whether the decision to admit someone to hospital was influenced by their social or other circumstances in addition to the severity of their condition.

Statistics are often quoted to show that women are more likely than men to be admitted to psychiatric hospitals or psychiatric wards of general hospitals. Table 2.14(b) shows that this was true of first admissions to mental-illness hospitals at all ages, except for children under 15, in 1976, but that the difference had disappeared for people under the age of 45 in 1986. The admission rate had dropped in all age groups except for men and women aged 75 and over, but it is not clear to what extent this decline had been offset by admissions to psychiatric units in district general hospitals, which are not included in these statistics.

In 1976, statistics about people living as long-stay patients in mental-illness hospitals, showed that, under the age of 65, men were more likely to do so than women. There are no corresponding statistics for 1986, but data should be available in the future through an annual census, linked to the Hospital Episode System, which will count the numbers of people who have been in hospital for more than a year.

It is hardly surprising that the numbers of people admitted to and living in long-stay hospitals have decreased, given the policy of closing them and replacing them by care given in district general hospitals and in the community. What is lacking, however, is adequate data to monitor the extent to which people are able to obtain the help and facilities they need to enable them to live outside long-stay institutions (Radical Statistics Health Group 1987).

The only routine data available about care outside hospital comes from the National Morbidity Surveys. Table 2.14(a) shows declining consultation rates attributed to 'mental disorder' over the ten years between the second and third survey in this series, but that from the age of 15 onwards, consultation rates remained higher for men than for women. It is difficult to tell to what extent this reflects higher rates of 'mental illness', or a greater likelihood of being diagnosed in this way by the rather atypical set of GPs who took part in the surveys.

Some of the points raised here were discussed in more detail in a study of apparent anomalies and reported differences between men and women in statistics on mental illness from Canada and the United States (Smith 1975). The author warned that 'the statistics on mental illness are put together as part of a system of professional and bureaucratic book keeping' and that additional meanings should not be read into them.

This warning applies more generally to the statistics discussed here. Despite their gaps, statistics about the provision of services are generally more plentiful, particularly at local level, than statistics about ill health, so it is tempting to use them as proxy measures, when in fact, they largely reflect the extent to which services are provided. Thus, for example, statistics about the whole-time equivalent numbers of home helps and the numbers of meals provided in people's own homes or in day centres are collected at local authority level, and show that provision rates vary very widely. On the other hand, statistics about the extent to which people have access to these services are collected through the General Household Survey which, because of the size of its sample, cannot be desegregated below regional level. It is therefore impossible to use them to look at variations in unmet need.

CONCLUSIONS

In broad terms, the conclusions to be drawn now are similar to those of a decade ago (Macfarlane 1980), but there are considerable differences in detail.

To start with the areas in which progress has been made, it is no longer true that the General Household Survey and the OPCS Longitudinal Study have been underused in analyses of women's health, and other chapters in this book bear witness to the extent to which they have been explored. This does not mean, of course, that the task is complete. There is still the potential to do more, both in terms of one-off analyses and in using the findings for monitoring trends over time.

There has also been considerable progress in collecting data about women's occupations and in classifying them in ways which can help to answer particular questions about the way women's work relates to their health. Here again, there is still more to be done to improve the completeness of the data and to tackle the technical problems of how to use information about the way women's employment interacts with childbearing and childrearing.

Table 2.14 Statistics of mental illness in men and women

a) People consulting GPs in selected practices and given a diagnosis of mental disorder (ICD 290–315), rates per 1000 population, England and Wales

	All ages	0–4	5–14	15–24	Age, years 25–44	45–64	65–74	75+
1971–2	(ICD 290–315)							
Male	73.6	58.6	37.2	58.4	91.2	95.1	71.3	75.7
Female	149.1	52.7	38.7	142.0	206.7	194.4	157.4	125.6
1981–2	(ICD 290–319)							
Male	55.4	36.6	17.5	37.9	64.8	77.7	69.7	91.2
Female	112.7	26.6	16.9	87.7	142.7	152.2	143.7	148.3

Source: Royal College of GPs, OPCS and DHSS, National Morbidity Survey, second and third national studies, 1974, 1986

b) First admissions to mental illness hospitals, rates per 100,000 population, England

	All ages	0–9	10–14	15–19	20–24	Age, years 25–34	35–44	45–54	55–64	65–74	75+
1976											
Male	104	9	23	80	142	139	133	116	104	142	351
Female	141	5	23	126	183	184	165	139	128	172	371
1986											
Male	100	10	24	65	114	118	104	87	89	114	411
Female	119	4	19	69	108	117	107	102	105	167	404

Source: Department of Health (1988) Health and Personal Services Statistics for England, 1988

c) People resident in mental illness hospitals on December 31st, rates per 100,000 population, England and Wales

| | All ages | 0–9 | 10–14 | 15–19 | Age, years | | | | | | | |
					20–24	25–34	35–44	45–54	55–64	65–74	75+
1976											
Male	159	4	12	28	65	95	135	246	332	417	608
Female	202	2	7	33	58	75	107	108	275	476	1035
1986				DATA NOT AVAILABLE							

Source: DHSS (1979). In-patient statistics from the Mental Health Enquiry, 1976

When it comes to statistics about health services, the news is less good, at least in England. The Steering Group on Health Services Information recommended a series of new data collection systems whose content was dominated by what were perceived to be the needs of administrators. Health authorities were then told, at a time of financial difficulty, to implement them within their existing financial resources. There has been wide variation in the extent to which they have succeeded or failed to implement the new systems, and thus aggregated national data are of questionable quality. In particular, national data have yet to emerge from the Hospital Episode System, which should cover all stays in NHS hospitals in England. Even more worrying is the possibility that, in the wake of the NHS white paper *Working for Patients* (Department of Health, Welsh Office, Northern Ireland Office and Scottish Office 1989), hospitals which opt out of health authority control may also opt out of national data collection systems (Freeman 1989), adding to the information gap which already exists in respect of private hospitals. It is to be hoped that the sorry tale of cervical cancer screening statistics will not be repeated in other contexts.

A positive step taken by the Department of Health is the requirement for district health authorities to monitor the health of their populations, and to reinstitute the annual report on the subject, which disappeared in the 1974 reorganization of the National Health Service and local government. While this is to be welcomed, it should be clear from what has been written here, that District Medical Officers, or Directors of Public Health as they are now to be known, will be hard put to find measures of morbidity and are thus likely to have to fall back, as in the past, on statistics of mortality and health service activity. Although the Department of Health announced that it was considering the feasibility of creating a 'health index' or portfolio of health indicators (Department of Health and Social Security 1988a), it did not publish its conclusions about what this might contain, or whether it was considered feasible to create one at all (Newton 1988). It would be very welcome if this initiative does lead to the collection of new morbidity data. This would be unlikely to be achieved without considerable cost as it would involve going out and surveying the population, locally as well as nationally.

One decision which has been made is to include a question

about chronic ill health in the 1991 census. Many problems were encountered when questions about particular 'infirmities' were asked in censuses from 1851 to 1911, after which the questions were abandoned (Macfarlane and Mugford 1984). In 1991, on the other hand, the question will be about long-term illness, and will thus be able to draw on experience in asking the similar question in the General Household Survey. It will be interesting to see what data emerge.

Considerations such as these are not, of course, peculiar to statistics about women, and some of the things which could be done to improve statistics about women would improve statistics about the population generally.

To return to the problems of women's health, Ann and Robin Oakley suggested that sexism may enter into the production of official statistics at the following levels:

> In the *areas* chosen for statistical analysis, in the *concepts* employed to organise and present the statistics, in the *collection* of data (including interactions between 'interviewer' and 'informant'), in the *processing* of statistics and in the *presentation* of the statistics.
>
> (Oakley and Oakley 1979)

Examples of all of these processes have been illustrated in this chapter. Despite the progress that has been made and the hope of future advances, some of the scope for further improvement is restricted by considerations which are not explicitly statistical, although they play a major role in shaping our statistics. First, definitions of such variables as 'head of household' reflect official perceptions of the current position of women in society and may not accurately describe the growing numbers of households which depart from these perceptions. Second, and more importantly in the context of statistics about health and illness, they are largely the product of the 'medical model' of health and illness. This tends to ignore the overwhelming importance of social and economic factors in the causation of illness and death. These factors can affect women in a different way than men, because of their different positions and roles in society. Alternatively, there is an increasing emphasis on measures of individual lifestyle factors associated with ill health, such as diet, smoking, and drinking. This is not be condemned in itself, but is unhelpful if it ignores the way they relate to the social and economic circumstances of women and men.

It would be unrealistic to expect official statistics of health and illness to do anything other than reflect the status quo. This means that more fundamental improvements in these statistics are unlikely to occur in the absence of changes in the prevailing view of the nature of health and illness. Thus it is not enough to devise technically more efficient ways of enumerating society, without also trying to change it.

ACKNOWLEDGEMENTS

Thanks to Lynda Pilcher for typing the tables in this paper and to Mel Bartley, Miranda Mugford, and other colleagues in the National Perinatal Epidemiology Unit and Karen Dunnell, Beverley Botting, and Laura Rodrigues for helpful comments on the contents.

NOTES

1. This chapter updates an earlier version written for the Social Science Research Council and the Equal Opportunities Commission (Macfarlane 1980). Thanks are again due to all the many people who contributed to the ideas in the original version.
2. Alison Macfarlane is funded by the Department of Health.
3. Crown Copyright is reserved.

Chapter Three

REVEALING WOMEN'S HEALTH: RE-ANALYSING THE GENERAL HOUSEHOLD SURVEY

SARA ARBER

Secondary analysis of the General Household Survey (GHS) provides enormous and largely untapped potential for addressing feminist issues about women's health. This chapter will briefly discuss the GHS and then illustrate some of the ways in which secondary analysis can be used to exploit GHS data. Three case-studies will illustrate different ways in which the GHS can be used for feminist analyses of health. The exemplars focus on gender differences in sickness absence, gender and care of elderly disabled people, and inequalities in women's health.

What is secondary analysis? Simply, it refers to any reworking of data which has already been analysed by some other researcher or organization (Dale *et al.* 1988). Hyman defines secondary analysis as 'any further analysis of an existing dataset which presents interpretations, conclusions or knowledge additional to, or different from, those presented in the first report on the inquiry' (Hyman 1972: 1). Because government data sets such as the GHS are relatively underanalysed by their originators, they provide a tremendous opportunity for secondary analysis.

The GHS is a multi-purpose continuous survey which has been carried out annually in Britain since 1971. It was designed to provide for the statistical needs of various government departments, for example: the Department of Health is concerned to monitor trends in the nation's health and use of health services; the Department of Employment is interested in trends in employment, unemployment, and patterns of job search; and the Department of the Environment uses the GHS to monitor migration and housing conditions. Other core areas asked about each year include education, income, family structure, and family formation. In addition, questions are asked about smoking and drinking every second year, and other topics covered at more irregular intervals include leisure activities, methods of family planning, the needs of the elderly, and incidence of burglaries. Good descriptive overviews of the GHS are provided in Bulmer (1986), Hakim (1982), and Dale *et al.* (1988). Because data are collected on a wide range of topics, the characteristics of women in each of these areas can be interlinked, perhaps in ways not considered by the sponsoring government departments, for example, smoking behaviour can be analysed according to women's class, employment status, housing tenure, quality of housing, family structure, and income.

The GHS is a large, nationally representative sample of private households. The sample contains about 10,000 households each year, and over 25,000 individuals. The response rate has varied between 80 per cent and 85 per cent in recent years. Further details about the sample design and response rates can be found in the GHS reports which are published annually. Each year, data is available on about 1,000 variables. Secondary analysis of GHS microdata is in some senses more akin to primary analysis, since the 200 pages of the GHS Annual Reports contain only a fraction of the possible analyses which could be performed on such a large data set containing so many variables. In addition, the annual reports present data in tabular form only, whereas secondary analysts can use more sophisticated multi-variate analyses and modelling techniques.

The large sample size of the GHS means reliable analyses can be conducted on proportionately small sub-groups in the population. For example, if a researcher wanted to study the health of women who have young children and who work full-time it would be difficult to obtain a representative sample, because such women form a small proportion of all women and there are no readily available sampling frames. However, by combining two or more years of GHS data together, a large enough sample is obtained to provide reliable estimates of their health and other characteristics, for example, whether their health differs from women in similar circumstances who are not in paid work or who work part-time.

The GHS is a household survey with a hierarchical structure. Comparable questions are asked of all adults in the household, and information is collected about the health and characteristics of all children under 16 years old. The amount of data collected for each household therefore varies in length depending on the number of families and number of persons in the household. Hierarchically organized surveys are extremely powerful data sources, allowing the researcher to address many theoretical questions not envisaged by the designer of the original survey. For example, Popay and Jones (1988) used secondary analysis of the GHS to study the health of children in the household and related this to the health of parents, and Payne (1987) analysed the relationship between the employment status of household members and showed the way in which unemployment seems to run in families. The ability to interrelate the characteristics of different individuals in the same household is a major advantage of secondary analysis of the GHS, although the conceptual and technical problems must not be under-estimated (Dale *et al.* 1988).

The GHS is available to researchers for secondary analysis in two forms (see Dale *et al.* 1988; chapter 5). It can be supplied by the ESRC Data Archive either as a flat SPSSX file based on individuals with information about the individual's household, housing, and the 'Head of Household' attached, or as a hierarchical file based on households. The latter contains records of varying length, depending on the number of individuals in the household, and must be analysed by a Database Management System such as SIR (Scientific Information Retrieval). SIR allows the researcher to analyse any of the interlinkages between individuals in the household which are present in the original GHS, but may not have been retained in the flat SPSSX files, for example, the smoking behaviour of spouses. A flat SPSSX file based on the GHS is relatively simple to analyse, once the researcher has obtained all necessary documentation and permission from the ESRC Data Archive, but the SIR GHS files are more complex than most novice users would wish to tackle. A full discussion of the alternative ways in which the GHS can be supplied, and of the process of ordering data sets from the ESRC Data Archive can be found in Dale *et al.* (1988).

The secondary analyst of the GHS need not be constrained to operate within the same set of conceptual assumptions as those held by the original designers. Clearly, the analyst is restricted by the questions which were asked in the GHS, and whole areas of relevance for a feminist analysis may have been omitted. However, analysts have some room for manoeuvre, because they may bring a totally different theoretical framework to bear on their research. For example, providing that sufficiently detailed information is collected about occupation and employment status, it is possible to re-analyse GHS data using different occupational classifications, which more adequately measure the distinctions between women's occupations (Dale *et al.* 1985). New household classifications can be devised which enable the study of the gender of co-resident carers, as discussed in the second case-study below, and the GHS may be used to compare 'conventional' approaches, which classify women according to their husbands' class, with an 'individualistic' approach, based on women's own occupation, as in the final case-study.

Many of the potential advantages of using the GHS for feminist analyses of health will be exemplified in the following three case-studies.

GENDER DIFFERENCES IN SICKNESS ABSENCE FROM WORK

The General Household Survey provides better statistics than those available from other data sources on gender differences in the level of sickness absence from work. This case-study relates to sickness absence before the introduction of the Statutory Sick Pay Scheme (SSP) in 1983.

Prior to 1983, the conventional source of information on gender differences in sickness absence was the National Insurance Sickness Absence statistics. These DHSS statistics showed that in 1979–80 married women had over 70 per cent more sickness absence than men, and non-married women had about 15 per cent more sickness absence than men.[1] However, these comparisons are biased because National Insurance (NI) statistics are based only on married women who paid the full National Insurance Contribution. At this time, about half of married women opted to pay a reduced rate National Insurance contribution and were therefore ineligible to claim sickness benefit on their own behalf. It is probable that women paying the full NI contribution were at greater risk of sickness and invalidity.

In 1982, the Equal Opportunities Commission (EOC) funded a study at the University of Surrey to examine gender differences in sickness absence based on secondary analysis of the 1975 and 1976 GHS (Dale *et al.* 1982; Allin *et al.* 1983). The particular interests of the EOC were twofold.

First, with the introduction of the Statutory Sick Pay Scheme (SSP) in 1983, employers were responsible for paying the first eight weeks of sickness benefit. The EOC were concerned that employers might assume that one sex generally had a worse record of sickness absence than the other, and that these erroneous assumptions might lead to discrimination in the employment of particular groups, such as working mothers with young children.

Second, there was evidence that insurance companies were charging an approximately 50 per cent higher premium for Permanent Health Insurance (PHI) for women than for men. The EOC wanted evidence from the GHS to argue that the statistical data on which these higher premiums were based was inadequate and that these insurance companies were in breach of Section 45 of the Sex Discrimination Act.

The GHS was chosen as an appropriate data source because it covered all employees and absences of all durations, therefore it did not suffer from the inadequacies of the National Insurance sickness absence statistics (OHE 1981). The GHS asked a question along the lines of 'were you away from work at all last week for reasons other than business?'. A subsequent question asked the reasons for this absence, and the focus here is on answers coded 'absence due to own illness or accident'. The analysis was based on men and women aged 18–60 who were working as employees in the week prior to the interview. The response rate in 1975 and 1976 was 84 per cent.

These analyses represent information on sickness absence for all employees, irrespective of entitlement to sickness benefit, working hours, or whether sickness absence is officially recorded by an employer. However, since the GHS data on sickness absence applies only to those who are in employment, it omits people who may have left the labour force because of long-term sickness. The fact that the GHS is a nationally representative sample means that findings for particular sub-groups can be expected to hold throughout Great Britain, and since interviewing is conducted evenly throughout the year, conclusions are not affected by seasonal fluctuations in illness.

Contrary to findings based on National Insurance records of

sickness absence claimants, the GHS shows little difference between men and women in the overall extent of sickness absence. Two contrasting trends are revealed, first, women report a some-what greater *frequency of spells* of sickness absence, but second, women are absent on average for a shorter *duration of time* than men. These contrasting trends are examined in Tables 3.1 and 3.2.

The frequency of spells of sickness absence is higher for women who work full-time (6.5 per cent report absence from work due to illness in the previous week) than for men (5.1 per cent report absence) – see Table 3.1 bottom line. A lower proportion of women who work part-time, 4.3 per cent, report absence due to sickness in the previous week.

Table 3.1 Percentage absent from work because of sickness in the previous week by whether has children under 16, working hours,* and sex

| | Women | | Men |
	Part-time	Full-time	Full-time
Has children	4.1%	6.8%	5.0%
N =	(2,675)	(1,404)	(6,479)
No children	4.6%	6.4%	5.3%
N =	(1,584)	(4,335)	(7,192)
Total	4.3%	6.5%	5.1%
N =	(4,259)	(5,739)	(13,671)
	5.5%		
	(9,998)		

Source: General Household Survey, 1975 and 1976 (author's analysis)
Note: * Full-time is defined as working for 30 or more hours a week.

Contrary to popular opinion, women with dependent children are no more likely to be away from work because of illness than women without children. Women who work full-time and have dependent children are very slightly more likely to report sickness absence than women without children, but among women working part-time the pattern is reversed (*see* Table 3.1)

Although there is evidence of higher frequency of spells of sickness absence for women working full-time than for men, the opposite is true for duration of absence. Table 3.2 shows that women are more likely than men to be absent for one to three days. There is a major gender difference for long periods of absence, 13 per cent of men had been absent for 41 or more days (over eight weeks) but this was the case for only half as many women, 7 per cent. The gender differential was even more marked for absences of over three months (66 days) – 8 per cent of men and 3 per cent of women who worked full-time. The finding that fewer full-time working women than men have long periods of sickness absence from work suggests that there is no evidence to support higher premiums for women for Permanent Health Insurance (PHI), which is the usual practice of insurance companies.

Table 3.2 Number of working days absent for this period of sickness by sex and working hours,* for employees absent through sickness during the previous week

| Days absent | Women | | Men |
| | Part-time | Full-time | Full-time |
	%	%	%
1–3 days	49	54	39
4–10 days	30	25	29
11–40 days	17	14	19
41 or more days	5	7	13
	100	100	100
N =	(181)	(367)	(695)

Source: General Household Survey, 1975–6 (author's analysis)
Note: * Full-time is defined as working for 30 hours or more a week.

A summary measure to compare gender differences in sickness absence is the average annual days of sickness absence from work, which takes into account *both* the frequency of absence (which is *higher* for women) and the duration of absence (which is *lower* for women). Women who work full-time have on average ten days sickness absence per year compared with nine days for men (see Table 3.3). This difference is substantially smaller than the figures suggested by the NI statistics reported earlier.

Analyses of the GHS also throw light on the main source of bias in NI statistics, which are based only on women who paid a full NI contribution. In the GHS, women who paid the full National Insurance contribution were more likely to be away from work in the previous week than those who were not eligible for sickness benefit – among women working full-time, 7.8 per cent and 5.8 per cent respectively. The differential was similar for women working part-time – 7.5 per cent of those paying the full NI contribution compared to 4 per cent who were paying the reduced rate.

Table 3.3 Average number of annual days of sickness absence from work by age group, for women and men working full-time

Age group	Women Full-time	Men Full-time	Women's number of absence days as a % of men's
18–24	9.3	8.1	115
N =	(1,529)	(2,144)	
25–34	11.0	7.7	143
N =	(1,129)	(3,637)	
35–44	11.9	8.2	145
N =	(1,141)	(3,057)	
45–54	8.5	11.4	75
N =	(1,391)	(3,171)	
55–60	11.2	10.9	103
N =	(547)	(1,655)	
All	10.1	9.1	111
N =	(5,737)	(13,662)	

Source: General Household Survey, 1975–6 (author's analysis)

Age is differently associated with the level of sickness absence for men and women. The extent of sickness absence broadly increases with age for men, the highest rates are for men over 45 years – approximately eleven days per year, compared with approximately eight days for men under 45 (Table 3.3). The pattern for women does not show a clear increase with increasing age, indeed women aged 45–54 report the lowest number of days absent. Although, overall, women working full-time have 11 per cent more absence days than men, in the 25–44 age group women have 40 per cent more absence days, whereas in the 45–54 age group women working full-time have a 25 per cent *lower* rate than men. These age differences may indicate that older women either leave the labour market or do not re-enter it if they are prone to illness.

Our analyses of sickness absence based on the GHS were used by the EOC in two ways. First, to dispel the myths about women having much higher rates of sickness absence than men; for example, leaflets were distributed in 1983 to employers pointing out the small gender differences in absence (Equal Opportunities Commission 1983). Second, the evidence on gender differences in length of illness is the opposite of what would be expected from the higher Permanent Health Insurance premiums for women. Since the GHS shows that men are much more likely to have been absent for long periods, this was used by the EOC as part of their evidence in a sex discrimination case against Friends Provident Insurance Company in 1983.[2]

GENDER DIFFERENCES AND CARE OF THE ELDERLY

A current policy concern is the needs of elderly people and, in particular, the rapidly increasing proportion of 'old' elderly, aged over 75, and over age 85 (Henwood and Wicks 1985). Provision for elderly people of health care and domiciliary support, both by the state and by the informal sector, are key areas of concern for policy analysts and feminists alike.

A number of small-scale, qualitative studies on care of the elderly graphically portray the burdens and sacrifices made by carers (Nissel and Bonnerjea 1982; Nissel 1984; Ungerson 1987; Wright 1983; Lewis and Meredith 1988). The carers in these studies were largely women, mainly because of the nature of the samples chosen for study, for example Nissel and Bonnerjea studied elderly people living with a married couple, and Lewis and Meredith's sample were daughters caring for an elderly parent. One result of these qualitative studies is that a popular image has been created that daughters perform the bulk of care for elderly disabled people, for example, Allan comments:

> Just as the bulk of housework and childcare is undertaken by mothers, so too by far the largest portion of routine tending for the elderly is provided by daughters . . . . The support at a daily level is almost wholly given by women and is defined as an extension of their routine domestic role.
>
> (Allan 1985: 130)

The General Household Survey is particularly valuable as a complement to small, qualitative, and localized studies. It provides a way of examining whether findings developed from smaller-scale research hold for a representative cross-section of the population.

It can therefore provide a means of testing theories and mapping the boundaries within which particular findings hold. The GHS, of course, cannot provide the wealth of detailed material about the meaning and experiences of caring, which can only be gleaned from more in-depth approaches to research.

The 1980 GHS provides a nationally representative sample of over 4,500 elderly people living in private households (OPCS 1982). People aged over 65 were asked a detailed section of questions on their ability to perform various activities of daily living, such as walking upstairs, doing shopping, and bathing themselves, and their use of various statutory health and welfare services in the previous month. The large sample size, high response rate (82 per cent), and representative nature of the sample therefore make the GHS a valuable data source to complement, extend, and systematically test findings and theoretical ideas derived from other small-scale studies. However, it is important to realize that the GHS is not representative of all frail elderly people because of the exclusion of those in institutional care.

This case-study uses the GHS to address two questions raised by feminists concerned about the care of the infirm elderly:

1 What is the sexual division of labour in caring for the infirm elderly?
2 Is there discrimination against women carers in the provision of statutory domiciliary services, such as home helps and district nursing care?

To answer these two questions it was necessary to develop an objective measure of the degree of disability of the elderly person. The assumption was that 'need' for support by a carer would be directly related to the elderly person's ability to manage activities of daily living on their own. A measure was constructed from a series of questions about the elderly person's ability to perform six daily tasks. These tasks formed a linear scale of increasing difficulty for most people: cutting one's toenails, getting up and down stairs, walking outside, bathing or washing all over, getting around the house, and getting in and out of bed (Arber *et al.* 1988). For each activity, the elderly person was given a score of 0 if they could perform the task easily on their own, a score of 1 if they could perform the task only with difficulty, and a score of 2 if the task could be done only with help or could not be done at all. 'Severe' disability was defined as a score of 6 or more on this scale. Elderly people who were 'severely' disabled needed assistance from one or more carers on a daily basis; they were unable to walk outside without help and most could not bath nor wash all over unaided.

Table 3.4 Percentage of elderly women and men with 'severe disability'* within age groups

| Age group | % with 'severe disability' | | | % of all with 'severe' disability |
	Women	Men	All	
65–69	5.5	3.7	4.7	16
70–74	8.5	7.2	8.0	21
75–79	12.6	9.0	11.3	21
80–84	25.8	17.2	22.5	21
85 and over	43.9	31.5	41.4	21
All	12.7	7.7	10.7	100
N =	(2,603)	(1,771)	(4,374)	(467)

Source: General Household Survey, 1980 (author's analysis)
Note: * 'Severe' disability is defined as a score of 6 or more, on a scale composed of the sum of scores on six activities of daily living. For each activity the score is 0 if the respondent can perform the activity easily, 1 if the elderly person performs the activity with difficulty, and 2 if the activity can only be done with help or by another person.

Table 3.4 shows that 10.7 per cent of people over age 65 are 'severely' disabled and need support on a daily basis. This varies from under 5 per cent of people in their late 60s to over 40 per cent of people aged over 85. More elderly women, 12.7 per cent, than elderly men, 7.7 per cent, are 'severely' disabled and in need of daily support. At each age, a higher proportion of women than men are in need of support. It is interesting to note that although the need for care increases very sharply with advancing age, the actual proportions of elderly people in need of daily support are approximately evenly distributed between the five age groups over 65 (see final column of Table 3.4).

Contrary to the impression from many smaller-scale studies, Table 3.5 shows that under a fifth of elderly people in need of daily support live with their children. These elderly people are almost equally divided between those living with an unmarried child and a married child. However, there is a marked gender difference between the carers in these two types of living arrangements.

About 40 per cent of disabled elderly people who live with an unmarried child are living with their son, but among comparable elderly people living with a married child other studies, such as Nissel and Bonnerjea (1982), suggest that the main carer is virtually always the woman.

Table 3.5 Living arrangements of (a) elderly people (age 65 and over) (b) 'severely' disabled elderly people, and (c) proportion of 'severely' disabled elderly people living with male carers

Type of household	(a) % of all elderly people	(b) % of all 'severely' disabled elderly people	(c) % with male co-resident carers*
Elderly living *Alone*	34	38	–
Elderly with *Spouse*:			
Couple only	46	31	51
Couple and adult children	6	6	28–84
Elderly with *Siblings* or other			
elderly	4	7	9–33
Elderly with *Unmarried Child*	6	9	38–45
Elderly with *Married Child*			
(and some lone parents)	4	8	0–5
	100	100	35–44
N =	(4374)	(467)	(288)

Source: General Household Survey, 1980 (author's analysis)

Note: * From the GHS it is not always possible to identify the gender of co-resident carers. In these cases, a range can be defined.

Nearly two-fifths of the elderly who need care on a daily basis live with their husband or wife. The GHS shows the perhaps surprising finding that equal numbers of men are caring for their wives as women are caring for their husbands. This confirms the findings of two EOC studies on carers (EOC 1980; Charlesworth *et al.* 1984). Among the 6 per cent of frail elderly living with their spouse and adult children, it is difficult from the GHS to identify the gender of the carer, because it is not clear whether the spouse or the younger person is the main carer. However, it is possible to define a range (*see* Table 3.5). A fuller discussion of the gender of carers of elderly disabled people is in Arber and Gilbert (1989a, 1989b).

Another category of carer which tends to be overlooked are the 7 per cent of elderly disabled people who live with other elderly people, generally their siblings. In these households, over two-thirds of carers are other elderly women.

A disadvantage of the 1980 GHS is that very little information is provided about the gender of informal carers who support the elderly living alone. Among the remainder of the elderly, Table 3.5 suggests that approximately 40 per cent of carers of the infirm elderly are men. This figure of 40 per cent male carers was confirmed in the 1985 GHS, which contained a section specifically designed to study informal carers (Green 1988). Such findings from large representative samples raise issues about why men have been neglected as carers. To what extent have men carers been neglected because they challenge dominant norms and values that caring is inherently feminine? In another paper (Arber and Gilbert 1989a), we suggest that men only take on the caring role when there has been a history of long-term co-residence with the elderly person. In these circumstances, there is generally a gradual change from a relationship of reciprocity to one of dependency. Women, unlike men, are also carers where an elderly person 'moves into' the household of the carer. They enter into caring relationships because of kinship obligations to care (Finch 1987). Research is needed to understand the similarities and differences between the caring trajectories of men and women, and to understand the circumstances under which men take on such intimate tasks as personal tending for the elderly. Thus, quantitative findings, such as these from the GHS, raise further questions which can be understood only by using more qualitative research methodologies.

The second issue of concern to feminists, which will be examined here, is that men carers receive more support from statutory services than women carers (Land 1978). The 1980 GHS provides evidence that discrimination is not primarily on the basis of gender alone, but is determined largely by the composition of the household in which the elderly person lives. Women carers are more likely to be in certain types of household which, on the whole, receive less service support. A range of domiciliary support services and personal health and social services was examined in Arber *et al.* (1988). The presentation of data here will be restricted to receipt of home helps and district nursing services in the last month.

In order to analyse discrimination in the receipt of services, it is necessary to control first for the elderly person's degree of disability. This is because the amount of support someone receives depends greatly on how well they can manage for themselves. The likelihood of an elderly person in different types of household receiving home helps and district nursing services is analysed by expressing the results as a comparison with a common standard.[3] For receipt of home helps, the standard is the likelihood of receipt by an elderly married couple, and for district nursing services, the standard is the likelihood of receipt by an elderly married man, where his wife is the main carer.

Figure 3.1a shows that, after controlling for level of disability, the major determinant of whether an elderly person receives a home help is the living arrangements of the elderly person. Elderly men and women who live alone are over five times more likely to receive home help support than an elderly married couple. An elderly person living with their unmarried son or daughter is less likely to receive a home help than an elderly married couple, but there is no apparent gender difference in home help provision where sons rather than daughters are carers. The group of elderly people least likely to receive home help support are those co-resident with a married couple – a living arrangement in which their daughter or daughter-in-law provides the bulk of their care.

Provision of district nursing care varies less (see Figure 3.1b), but the major determinant of service receipt is the type of household of the elderly person rather than the gender of carer. Disabled women cared for by their husbands are about 20 per cent more likely to receive district nursing support than where a disabled husband is cared for by his wife. Similarly, unmarried sons who care for an elderly parent are about 20 per cent more likely to receive district nursing care than unmarried daughters. Elderly disabled people living with a married child receive the least district nurse support. It is clear that the substitution of informal carers for statutory domestic and personal health services is greater where women are carers. However, this occurs not primarily because of discrimination against women *per se* but because of discrimination against particular types of household and types of caring relationship in which women predominate as carers, especially where there are married women under 65 in the household. These analyses show that it is the family, and especially married women, who bear a large proportion of the costs of dependency.

Figure 3.1 Receipt of home helps and district nursing care in the last
month by living arrangements of the elderly person,
controlling for disability, odds ratios

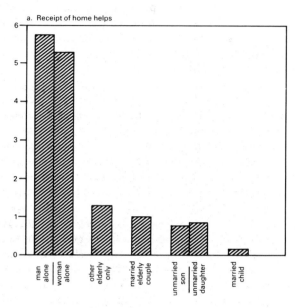

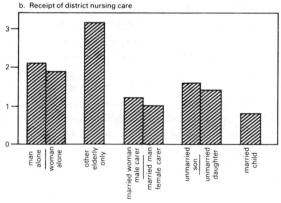

Source: General Household Survey 1980 (author's analysis)

Domestic and personal health service receipt is thus dependent not only on the physical needs of the elderly person, but also on the assessment of the ability or perceived willingness of the carers to provide these services themselves. Although the GHS cannot be used to provide evidence of direct discrimination against certain categories of carer, it provides evidence of the disadvantaged position of married women who are co-resident with elderly disabled people.

INEQUALITIES IN WOMEN'S HEALTH

The third case-study will illustrate how large-scale data from the GHS can contribute to our understanding of inequalities in women's health. The major concern of the Black Report (DHSS 1980) was inequalities in men's health. Since its publication, a growing number of studies have examined inequalities in women's health. However, these studies present largely contradictory findings because of a failure to conceptualize adequately the socio-economic circumstances of women. The *Health Divide* (Townsend *et al.* 1988) reviewed evidence on gender and health and concluded 'all in all, these studies raise more questions than answers and the whole field is ripe for further research' (p. 245) . . . 'research is only just beginning to unravel the complexities of inequality in health for women' (ibid. 1988: 255). This case-study will address some aspects of this complexity and provide a clearer framework for understanding inequalities in women's health. Two particular concerns will be (1) are there as strong class differences for women as for men? and (2) whether different theoretical models are required to understand inequalities in short-term illness (health state) compared to longer term health problems (health status).

Using secondary analysis researchers can analyse data in very different ways from the approaches used in published reports. They need not be 'hidebound' by government (official) assumptions about the appropriate way to classify women (Oakley and Oakley 1979). This case-study therefore illustrates the advantages of secondary analysis of survey microdata rather than relying solely on published tables from the GHS.

The health tables in the GHS annual reports classify women according to their husband's occupation if they are married, and all other women by their own current occupation (or last occupation if they are not working) (OPCS 1989a). This approach has been strongly criticized by feminists (Stanworth 1984; Allen 1982), but defended by others, such as Goldthorpe (1983, 1984). It has come to be known as the 'conventional' approach. Many feminists argue that women should not be characterized as dependent on their husbands but should be classified by their own occupation – using an 'individualistic' approach. Secondary analysis of the GHS allows an assessment of these two approaches to understanding class inequalities in women's health, which cannot be done solely from tables in the published GHS reports.

The data presented in this case-study are based on women aged 20–59 in the 1981 and 1982 GHS. Two years of GHS data have been combined to provide a larger sample and therefore more reliable estimates for proportionately small sub-groups, such as divorced, separated, and widowed women.

When analysing inequalities in women's health it is helpful to consider differences between various measures of health, and to theorize how they relate to class and to women's domestic and employment roles. Blaxter (1985) distinguishes between indicators of temporary health state – 'Am I ill today?' – which represent the present state of health of the individual, and indicators of longer term health status – 'Am I a basically healthy or unhealthy person?' – which provides a more general characteristic. Health state is similar to, but not the same as, acute illness and health status is related to, but not the same as, chronic illness. Although health state is a more erratic condition than health status, they are related, since health state may be a consequence of health status, and health state may be reflected back to be incorporated in health status. This case-study illustrates Blaxter's distinction by using two health measures derived from the GHS:

Limiting long-standing illness (LLI) is a measure of *health status* which is related to function. In the GHS the respondent was asked, 'Have you any long-standing illness, disability or infirmity?' If the answer was 'Yes', the respondent was then asked whether it limited his or her activities in any way (OPCS 1984a). This measure represents the consequences of health status for what the individual perceives as his or her 'normal' activities. It represents a self-assessment of the effect of any chronic ill health on daily life.

Restricted activity (RA) days due to illness reported in the previous two weeks is a measure of *health state,* based on the individual's perception of whether symptoms have altered their 'normal' activities over a specified time period. The proportion of women who report restricted activity will be used, as well as a variable measuring the average number of restricted activity days in a year. The latter is derived by multiplying the number of restricted activity days in a two-week period by 26.

Table 3.6 Measures of ill health by age for women (age 20–59)

	20–29	30–39	40–49	50–59	Total
(a) Longstanding illness					
– limits activities	8	13	18	26	16
– non-limiting	9	12	14	15	12
– no long-standing illness	82	76	68	59	72
	100	100	100	100	100
N =	(3,842)	(3,999)	(3,244)	(3,411)	(14,496)
(b) Restricted activity					
% reporting restricted activity in last 14 days	11.5	11.2	13.6	13.4	12.3
Restricted activity days in last year	19	20	25	29	23
N =	(3,841)	(3,997)	(3,241)	(3,411)	(14,490)

Source: General Household Survey, 1981–2 (author's analysis)

Both health status and health state are associated with age. Table 3.6a shows that a higher proportion of older women report a limiting long-standing illness, 26 per cent of women in their fifties, compared with 8 per cent of women in their twenties. Non-limiting long-standing illness increases less steeply with age from 9 per cent of women in their twenties to 15 per cent of women in their fifties. The following analyses are restricted to limiting long-standing illness. Health state varies less with age; 11 per cent of women under 40 report illness which restricted their activity in the previous two weeks, which increased to only 13 per cent for women over 40 (Table 3.6b). However, when the average number of restricted activity days per year is examined, the age trend becomes clearer, varying from 18 days for women in their twenties up to nearly 30 days for women in their fifties.

Factors influencing women's health status

Prior to embarking on secondary analysis of survey data, it is important to have a clear model of the relationships between relevant variables. Figure 3.2 presents a simple model of the key factors associated with poor health status. The analysis here will focus only on some of the components of this model. Such a model will help in understanding the reasons for different findings when using a 'conventional' versus an 'individualistic' approach to class analyses of women's health status.

Figure 3.2 Key variables associated with health status

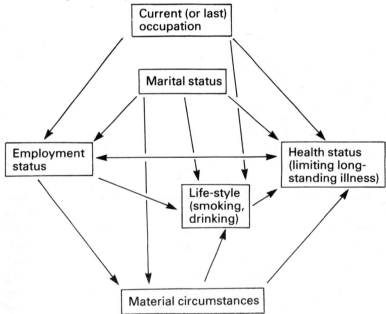

Since age is closely related to health status (Table 3.6), it is essential to remove any effects of age when analysing the relationship between a woman's class and her health status. For example, if some classes contain proportionately more older

81

women and women in these classes have poorer health, this might
be a spurious effect caused by their older average age. Analyses of
mortality usually remove the potentially spurious effects of age by
calculating Standardized Mortality Ratios (SMRs), as has been
done in the chapter by Pugh and Moser in this book (chapter 4).
SMRs are a way of comparing the mortality of different groups with
a standard of 100, which represents the mortality of all women.
The same procedure can be used for analysing any measure of
health, such as limiting long-standing illness. In this case-study,
differences in age structure between each group are removed by
using the indirect method of standardization to calculate
Standardized Limiting Long-standing Illness (SLLI) Ratios, using
10-year age bands.

For analyses of women's class and health the ideal would be to
use a measure which more sensitively captures distinctions
between women's occupations (Abbott and Sapsford 1987; Arber
et al. 1986; Dale *et al.* 1985), but the secondary analyst is restricted
to the variables and coding categories available in the data set.
Between 1977 and 1984 the GHS did not code detailed information about the individual's occupational unit group, so
during these years it was impossible to derive variables which more
adequately measured women's occupational class. The class
measure used in the GHS is a categorization of the Registrar
General's Socio-Economic Groups (SEG). This is similar to the
familiar Registrar General's social classes, but has a number of
differences, especially for women's occupations (Arber *et al.* 1986).
The GHS 'collapsed' SEG will be used here with a minor
modification to separate out women working in semi-professional
occupations, such as nursing and teaching (SEG 3a), from women
working in intermediate and junior non-manual occupations (SEG
3b).

For men there is a strong class gradient with limiting long-
standing illness (standardized to remove the effects of age
differences between classes) (see Figure 3.3c). This linear class
gradient is very similar to the mortality gradient for men (OPCS
1986a). Unskilled men have a very disadvantaged health status –
they report 55 per cent more limiting long-standing illness than
the national average, while professional men have 34 per cent less
long-term illness than all men (Arber 1989).

Figure 3.3 Standardized limiting long-standing illness ratios by class for women and men (20–59) age standardized

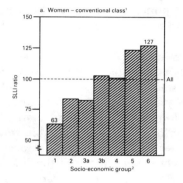

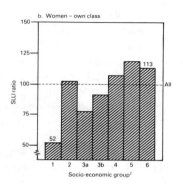

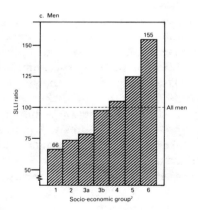

Source: General Household Survey, 1981–2 (author's analysis)

Notes: [1] Women with husbands are classified by their husbands' occupation, women of other marital statuses are attributed to their own (current or last) occupational class.
[2] *Socio-economic group*
1 Higher professional, 2 Employers and managers, 3a Lower professional, 3b Supervisory and junior non-manual, 4 Skilled manual and own account, 5 Semi-skilled manual and personal services, 6 Unskilled manual

The class gradient for women using the 'conventional' approach (Figure 3.3a) is similar to men, but the disadvantaged position of women classified as 'unskilled' is less pronounced than for unskilled men (27 per cent more 'unskilled' women have a long-standing illness than all women). The gradient is not entirely linear, since women classified as 'junior non-manual' have an equivalent level of chronic illness to those in the 'skilled manual' category.

Characterizing women by their own occupation, an 'individualistic' approach, no longer produces a straight-line relationship but is curvilinear (Figure 3.3b). The small number of women with professional occupations have a very advantaged health status, 48 per cent fewer have a limiting long-standing illness than all women. But, women who are 'employers and managers' have a poorer health status than other women in non-manual occupations and than men in the same class. This illustrates the way in which the same class may have different effects for women and men. The 'individualistic' approach shows only minor differences in health status among women working in the three manual classes. Women's manual occupations may have different meanings in terms of skill level and relative standing compared with the class distinctions conventionally drawn between men's occupations (Dex 1984). These different patterns for women's own occupations raise questions. There is a need to analyse the pattern for women in their own right, rather than holding it up to the male standard and treating any differences between the patterns for women's and men's occupations as an anomaly. Analyses which present smaller class differences for women are in danger of interpreting this as evidence of reflecting less inequality in society for women than for men, rather than the occupational inadequacy of the tools used to measure women's class (Arber 1990).

Our understanding of the different relationships between class and health in Figure 3.3 can be advanced only from an appreciation of the wider network of factors influencing health status described in Figure 3.2. A distinction which is often not explicitly recognized in studies of women's health is that class is used to measure two conceptually distinct aspects of material explanations of inequalities in health. First, the material circumstances of the woman's household influences her health, and second, the nature of her paid employment may have a direct influence on her health. For men, these two aspects of material position work in concert to increase inequalities in health, since a man's occupation is assumed to be both a primary determinant of his material circumstances, and has a direct bearing on his health.

Greater class inequalities in health status are found for men than women probably because a man's occupational class provides a better measure of his household's material circumstances than is the case for women, and material conditions are the major factor influencing health status. Women's health status measured by the 'conventional' approach (classifying married women by their husband's occupation and other women by their own current or last occupation) shows a pattern which is similar but weaker than for men.

It is perhaps naïve to expect that a married woman's own occupational class would have as profound an influence on her health as is the case for a man. There may be some direct effect of her own paid employment on her health, but the major effect of material conditions is likely to be better captured by other measures of the material circumstances of that woman. In analysing men's health, a man's occupational class can be used as a surrogate for both the material conditions extant in his household and the direct effects of the nature of paid employment on his health. For women, it is necessary to separately theorize and measure the effects of a woman's material circumstances from any effects of her own employment status and the nature of her own occupation.

Although the 'conventional' way of measuring class for women shows a stronger association with poor health status than the 'individualistic' approach, it is conceptually complex because it combines two gender-differentiated occupational structures. Married women are assigned to the male occupational structure, which places more men in the higher reaches of both the non-manual and manual segments of the labour market. Single and previously married women are categorized by their own occupation and therefore assigned disproportionately to the lower reaches of the class structure (Martin and Roberts 1984). In the 'conventional' approach a woman's marital role is the sole criterion for deciding which gender-segregated class structure to use. Therefore, it is important to understand the ways in which marital status itself is associated with health status.

Married women have much better health status than single or previously married women – 7 per cent fewer married women report limiting long-standing illness than the average for all women (the SLLI Ratio is 93 for married women). Single women have a poorer health status – 18 per cent more report long-standing illness than all women. Women who are divorced, separated, or widowed have the poorest health status; 40 per cent more have a limiting long-standing illness than all women. The direction of influence between marital status and poor health is not entirely clear; poor health status may be a disadvantageous factor in the marriage and remarriage markets. To understand the implications of using the 'conventional' approach when analysing inequalities in women's health, it is helpful to analyse separately class differences in health status for married, single, and previously married women (Figure 3.4).

Married women, irrespective of their class, have relatively good health status (Figure 3.4a and 3.4b). However, the effects of a woman's own occupation on her health are very considerable for single and previously married women (Figure 3.4c and 3.4d). For these women, the major health disadvantage is experienced by women working in manual occupations, who are over 50 per cent more likely to have a limiting long-standing illness than all women. Single women in non-manual occupations have as good health status as equivalent married women.

The occupational class of single women reflects both the direct effects of occupation and the effects of material circumstances in the same way as for men, but this is not the case for married women. The particularly poor health status of previously married women needs detailed research, in particular the direction of causality of the relationship. Previously married women are more likely to live in poor material circumstances, because their earnings are often insufficient as a 'family wage'. Lone mothers are particularly likely to be reliant on state benefits (Glendinning and Millar 1987)

If this case-study were to be extended it would need to take into account whether women are in paid employment, since housewives are more likely to be in poor health (Arber 1987), and how to measure more adequately material conditions for women (Arber 1990). The ideal would be a multi-variate analysis of all the variables in Figure 3.2, including lifestyle variables, such as smoking and drinking.

Factors influencing women's health state

The factors which influence women's health state are likely to differ from those influencing health status in two important respects. First, health status influences health state. The main reason for the increase in poor health state with age is because age brings long-term illness. Second, the combination of women's employment, parental, and marital roles may result in role stress, which in turn influences the woman's health state. But the resulting level of role stress will vary with the woman's structural position. Women in disadvantaged material circumstances may be less likely to be able to cope with the stresses of being a mother and full-time employee than women in more 'privileged' circumstances. The extent to which partners contribute to the domestic division of labour will influence a woman's ability to manage the demands of fulfilling a number of roles, and their likelihood of role overload and poor health state. Figure 3.5 provides an outline model of the key structural and role-related factors associated with health state. All these variables, except equality of the domestic division of labour, could be analysed using the GHS.

An earlier study using the 1975–6 GHS examined two contrasting theses that (a) paid employment has beneficial effects on women's health state through role accumulation, and (b) that paid employment has adverse consequences due to role strain (Arber *et al* 1985). This study found adverse health consequences for women with children, who work full-time in lower non-manual and in manual occupations. The picture was somewhat different for women with professional and managerial jobs. Their greater financial resources could be used to ease some of the burdens of housework and childcare, so reducing role strain and fatigue. In addition, women working full-time in professional and managerial occupations are likely to have more flexible hours and more control over their work, making it easier to fit in with the demands of children, compared with women in lower level jobs who have less autonomy and more rigid work schedules. Thus, the adverse consequences of occupying the roles of mother,

Figure 3.4 Standardized limiting long-standing illness ratios by class and marital status for women (20–59), age standardized

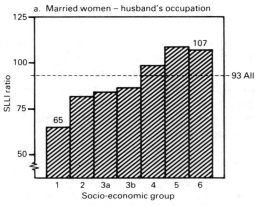

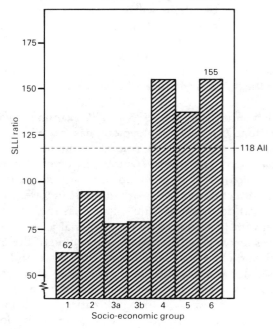

Figure 3.4 continued Standardized limiting long-standing illness ratios by class and marital status for women (20–59), age standardized

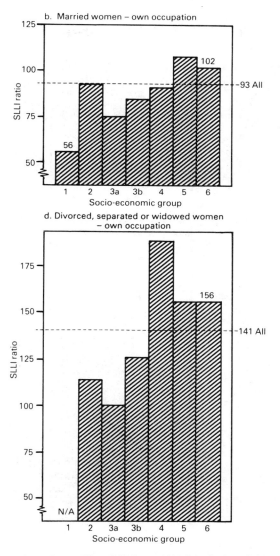

Source General Household Survey, 1981–2 (author's analysis)

Note: * Class is coded into socio-economic groups as in Figure 3.3 (*See* p. 83)

Figure 3.5 Key factors associated with health state among women
(restricted activity due to illness)

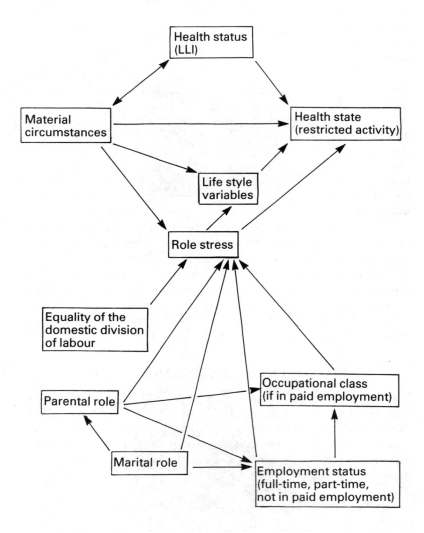

housewife, and full-time worker are less for women in more 'privileged' structural positions. Indeed there may be positive benefits of role accumulation for these women. For other women freedom to work may be a dubious freedom if it means that they have little time to do anything except paid work, unpaid domestic tasks, and routine childcare.

Analyses of the health state of women must therefore consider the strain many women face in maintaining multiple roles as full-time employees, mothers, and housewives. Adverse health effects are likely to be mediated if there is greater equality in the domestic division of labour, but most evidence at present points in the direction of increased labour force participation for women with children but little change in traditional gender roles in the home (Martin and Roberts 1984). Women need to have a basically good health status in order to contemplate the rigours of coping with paid employment, childcare, and the housewife role.

These three case-studies exemplify a number of different ways in which the GHS can be fruitfully analysed to throw light on key areas of concern for feminists interested in women's health. Data collection is an expensive exercise, and prohibitively so for researchers on the scale available through the GHS. The GHS provides a large body of high quality data, which to date has been underexploited. This resource could well be used more fully, as these examples serve to demonstrate.

ACKNOWLEDGEMENTS

I would like to thank the Office of Population Censuses and Surveys for permission to use the General Household Survey, and the ESRC Data Archive, University of Essex for supplying the data. I am very grateful to my colleagues Angela Dale and Nigel Gilbert, who were co-researchers on much of the work discussed in this paper.

1. See Table A of Allin *et al.* (1983). This Table was derived from Table D2 in the Report of the Government Actuary on the First Quinquennial Review under section 137 of the Social Security Act 1975, 'National Insurance Fund, Long Term Financial Estimates', House of Commons paper 451, July 1982, HMSO.
2. The case of Pinder versus Friends Provident Insurance Company was contested between 1983 and 1985, but was unsuccessful in the courts.

3. A logit analysis was carried out using GLIM with receipt of services as the dependent variable and type of household and level of disability as the independent variables. The odds ratios in Figure 3.1 are derived from the coefficients of a main effects logit model.

Chapter Four

MEASURING WOMEN'S MORTALITY DIFFERENCES

HELENA PUGH AND KATH MOSER

In our everyday lives we observe huge health inequalities all around us. When walking down the street, travelling on a bus, or shopping in a supermarket we see evidence of health differences. By using statistics we are able to study aspects of these health differences systematically and to help answer important questions such as: How large are the health inequalities? Does poor health affect a tiny group or a large proportion of the population? How are inequalities changing over time? Statistics can be used to provide concrete evidence of health inequalities and therefore prevent the dismissal of our everyday observations as anecdotal. They provide a basis from which to formulate social policy, and place us in a stronger position to campaign for better health for all.

Recent years have seen a growing interest in the nation's health with particular emphasis on social inequalities, i.e., the difference in health and quality of life experienced by those at the bottom of the social scale from those at the top (Townsend *et al.* 1988; Smith and Jacobson 1988). Women's health has received relatively little consideration compared to that given to men. Emphasis has been on investigating men's morbidity and mortality according to their social circumstances (usually measured by their occupation or social class). For example, men in manual occupations have higher mortality in the working age range than those in non-manual occupations (Fox and Goldblatt 1982). However, using occupation as an indicator of social classification has considerable problems when analysing data concerning women. In this chapter we focus on women's mortality and begin by discussing the problems and issues of using occupation in the social classification of women. We suggest an alternative approach which is more appropriate to women's lives. Using routinely collected statistics we investigate mortality differences and consider whether a combination of indicators provides a better measure of the social circumstances of women than does occupation alone.

NEGLECT OF WOMEN (AND MORE SPECIFICALLY WOMEN'S INTERESTS) IN STUDIES OF MORTALITY AND SOCIAL CLASSIFICATION

There are two important reasons for the lack of attention to social class differences in women's mortality. First, there has been a well-documented lack of attention to women, and issues specifically relating to women, in all academic disciplines. This includes epidemiology. Second, and related to the first problem, are the particular difficulties associated with satisfactorily analysing women's mortality data by occupation. Hard though it may be to consider women's mortality in relation to their social class, if the difficulties had pertained to men's mortality researchers would by now undoubtedly have found a way!

Problems with using own occupation as a measure of social position

Using occupation as a measure of social position is intended to provide a rough indicator of a person's standard of living, way of life, and command over resources. The lesser importance given to women's jobs as compared to men's, the assumption that breadwinners are male, that women are dependent on men, and that women's role is primarily that of homemaker, all contribute to the many problems associated with using own occupation to classify women.

Although most women are in employment for much of their working lives, at any one point in time a large proportion are housewives. The 1971 Census found that 53 per cent of women in the 'working' age range 15–59 could be classified to an occupation and hence a social class (see Figure 4.1). The remaining 47 per cent of women who could not be classified to an occupation were mainly housewives. We use 1971 to illustrate the points we wish to make as the data source we are working with is based on a sample from the 1971 Census.

Figure 4.1 Distribution of women aged 15–59 in 1971 by own social class

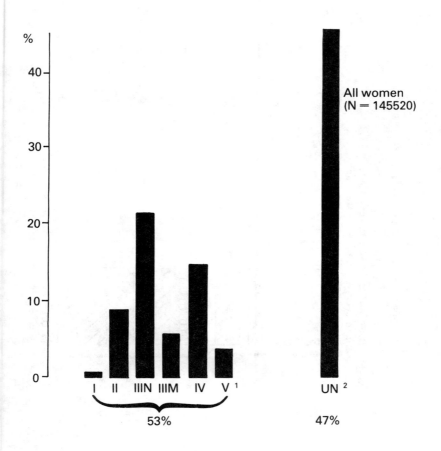

Source: OPCS Longitudinal Study (authors' analysis)
Notes: [1] I to V: social classes
[2] UN: unclassified (housewives, students, permanently sick or disabled,
inadequately described occupations, armed forces).
© Crown Copyright

Figure 4.2 Distribution of women aged 15–59 in 1971 with an occupation by occupation unit

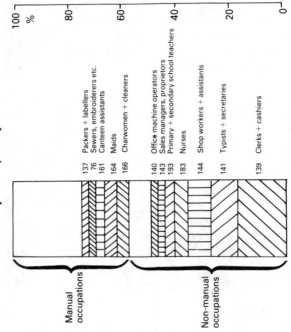

Source: OPCS Longitudinal Study (authors' analysis)
© Crown Copyright

The problems with using occupation are particularly acute in mortality studies as even fewer women have an occupation recorded on their death certificate than on the census schedule. This stems from the instructions given to Registrars concerning occupational recording at death, which emphasize the recording of husband's occupation for married women. Only for women in full-time work at death is much attempt made to record own occupation; part-time work is disregarded as is previous full-time work unless the woman has been in paid employment for most of her life. Consequently in 1970–2 own occupation was recorded for only 20 per cent of the deaths to women aged 15–64; the proportion was much lower among married and widowed women (10 per cent and 12 per cent respectively) than among single women (72 per cent) (Office of Population Censuses and Surveys 1978a).

For those women who can be classified to a social class using occupation there are additional problems. The Registrar General's occupational classification does not differentiate adequately between the jobs that most women do. In 1971 half the women who could be classified to an occupation fell into just six (of more than 200) occupation units (see Figure 4.2). Most women were in Social Classes IIIN (clerks, secretaries, shop assistants, etc.) and IV (canteen assistants, maids, charwomen, etc.), and to a lesser extent Social Class II (teachers, nurses, etc.).

Finally, using a woman's own occupation as a sole measure of her social position is problematic because employment experiences differ greatly according to marital status (see Figure 4.3). In the age range 15–59, 69 per cent of single women could be allocated to a social class in 1971 as compared to 47 per cent of married women. Conversely, over 50 per cent of married women were not classified to an occupation (predominantly housewives) while this was the case for only about 30 per cent of single women (predominantly schoolgirls and students).

This evidence confirms that women's employment patterns are strongly related to their marital status; this is largely because of childcare responsibilities. Women's moves in and out of the labour force relate to their domestic responsibilities such as caring for children, elderly relatives and other dependants, husbands, and homes. Consequently, many married women work part-time (49 per cent of those in employment in 1971), and many women do

Figure 4.3 Distribution of single and married women aged 15–59 in 1971 by own social class

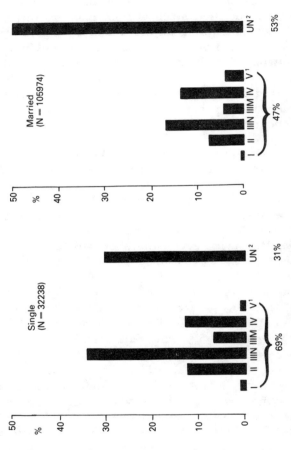

Source: OPCS Longitudinal Study (authors' analysis)

Notes: [1] I to V: social classes

[2] UN: unclassified (housewives, students, permanently sick or disabled, inadequately described occupations, armed forces).

© Crown Copyright

paid work at home or work split shifts. Since jobs are taken to fit round other commitments, women's occupations do not reflect their skills, training, or full potential; this situation is compounded by sex discrimination in the labour market. A recent analysis (Dex 1987) from the Women and Employment Survey shows that downward occupational mobility often occurs after childbearing; this reflects both a lack of job opportunities for women with children and a lack of good childcare facilities. All these factors lead us to conclude that women's lives cannot be summed up by their paid employment alone.

The traditional approach – use of husband's occupation

The approach most frequently used by researchers and government statisticians to classify women has been to use own occupation until marriage and from then onwards to use husband's occupation. This is the approach taken by the Decennial Supplements on mortality (OPCS 1978a, 1986a) which provide the main source of information on socio-economic differentials in mortality for England and Wales. They present mortality data calculated using deaths around the time of the census to the corresponding population at census. As this method requires the comparison of information from death registration and census, it is limited to information which can be reliably obtained from both sources which, in effect, means occupation. As a result of the lack of occupational information at death for women, husband's occupation is usually used to classify married women, own occupation for single and divorced women, and either own or husband's for widowed women.

Problems with using husband's occupation for married women

Classifying women using husband's occupation has serious limitations. There are many objections (Delphy 1981) including the ideological (that it is offensive to describe women solely in terms of their husband's occupation), and the logical (that it ignores aspects of women's own lives). Using only husband's occupation disregards other material circumstances which we imagine to be important to women's lives, such as their own employment position and occupation, their work in the home, i.e., domestic responsibilities, and the contribution their own earnings make to their households' standard of living.

Meaningful comparisons between women of different marital statuses are impossible if married women are only classified by their husband's occupation. In addition, this method does not provide a direct means of examining the effect of a married woman's own occupation on her health. Research has clearly established links between specific occupations and particular causes of death (OPCS 1978a; Goldblatt *et al.* forthcoming). In particular the Longitudinal Study (LS) has been used to investigate women's mortality using their own occupation and has suggested, for example, that mortality from heart disease is high amongst cooks (Moser and Goldblatt in preparation).

AN ALTERNATIVE APPROACH

A more wide-ranging study of mortality differentials among women than has been previously possible can be carried out using data from the OPCS Longitudinal Study (LS). Although it was not custom-made to answer our specific questions, it does provide a valuable opportunity for studying women's mortality. The LS is a prospective study of a 1 per cent sample of the population of England and Wales enumerated at the 1971 Census. It links the census information on individuals to their death records in subsequent years. By following up individuals from the census, the LS enables us to consider mortality differences using the socio-economic information collected at census. Hence we are able to classify a far greater percentage of women to an occupation than can be achieved using occupation at death; this makes mortality analyses by social class more feasible.

However, as we have seen, there are problems associated with using occupation alone. A further advantage of the LS is that we can analyse mortality according to other socio-economic characteristics, in particular housing tenure (owning or renting your house) and household access to cars, which have been used successfully elsewhere as proxies for social class (Fox and Goldblatt 1982; Arber 1989). Here we have used these household characteristics in conjunction with economic activity (in paid employment or not) and own and husbands' social class. Housewives, in particular, can therefore be classified in terms of a broader view of their socio-economic circumstances than their husbands' jobs alone. While feeling that it is inappropriate to judge a woman's life chances entirely on the social class of her husband, women are clearly affected by the social standing of their husbands, even if they do not always share the same standard of living (Graham 1984). As domestic responsibilities are central to women's lives we have also considered whether a woman is working full- or part-time and if she has dependent children in her household.

Methods

We have looked at the relationship between mortality from all causes and socio-economic circumstances at the time of the 1971 Census. Further information about the LS and the methods used is given elsewhere (Fox and Goldblatt 1982; OPCS 1988c). We have restricted our analysis to women in the 'working' age range (15–59). We have concentrated on mortality in the period 1976–81; deaths in the first few years after the census were affected by health selection processes, which become less important over time (Fox *et al.* 1982a; Fox *et al.* 1985). The healthy worker effect is the health selection process most frequently mentioned. This is

... the common finding ... that people at work have lower mortality rates than the rest of the population ... You should not be confused into thinking that this low mortality demonstrates the beneficial effect of work. It can usually be shown that it is a direct result of the selection processes which determine who gets jobs and who loses jobs. However, in some cases it may reflect, for example, the beneficial effect involved in work, leading to a reduction in the risk of, say, heart attacks.

(Fox *et al.* 1982b: 14)

Another example of health selection is that single women are often found (as here) to have higher mortality than married women, and this can be largely attributed to health selection. A sizeable proportion of those women who remain single suffer from some physical or mental disability or illness (Kiernan 1988).

As a result of the very different lifestyles of single and married women we have considered these groups separately; women separated from their husbands were classified as married by the

1971 Census. Few women (5 per cent) aged 15–59 were widowed or divorced in 1971 and they were excluded from our analysis. (Widowhood is not common in this age range, and in 1971 divorce was infrequent as the 1969 Divorce Reform Act had only just come into effect.) All the women were grouped according to their economic activity, own social class (measured by occupation), housing tenure, and whether their household had access to a car. The information on cars was obtained from the 1971 Census question:

> How many cars and vans are normally available for use by you or members of your household (other than visitors)?

For married women, husbands' social class was also included in the analysis. Information on occupation was obtained from 1971 Census questions on economic activity which were asked:

> in respect of the main employment last week, or of the most recent job if retired or out of work. For persons who have never had a job and for a housewife who did not have a job last week, write 'NONE'.

Using this information women were allocated to the Registrar General's Social Classes. Married women who could be allocated to an occupation (on the basis of their current or most recent job) were considered separately from those who were housewives.

Finally for married women we have considered whether those in paid employment were working full- or part-time; in line with the definition used in many official surveys women working 30 hours or less were classified as part-time workers. As an indicator of their domestic responsibilities, we also considered whether they had a dependent child (defined as under 17 years). The 1971 Census fertility questions referred to legitimate births and were only asked of ever-married women; therefore our information about dependent children is restricted to this group. However since single parenthood was uncommon in 1971 this is unlikely to be a significant problem in our analysis.

Standardized mortality ratios (SMRs) were used as summary indices of mortality. An SMR compares the total number of deaths observed among a group of people with the number expected in a population of the same size and age structure; the expected deaths are calculated using death-rates in a reference population. Here the reference population is all women in the LS and the groups we have concentrated on are subsets of this larger group. The SMR is calculated by multiplying the ratio of observed to expected deaths by 100; hence, an SMR over 100 indicates a level of mortality higher than that of the reference group, and an SMR less than 100 suggests lower mortality. For example, women classified as 'Engineering and allied trades workers not elsewhere classified' had an SMR of 129, i.e. high mortality, while those who were 'Professional, technical workers and artists' had low mortality with an SMR of 69 (Moser and Goldblatt in preparation). Tests of statistical significance (confidence intervals – CI) were performed to assess whether the seemingly high (or low) mortality arose by chance, or whether we can be reasonably confident that it is a meaningful finding. By presenting the 95 per cent CIs we indicate that there is only a 5 per cent probability of the 'true' value of the SMR lying outside this interval. Hence a 95 per cent CI, which excludes 100, provides strong evidence that the mortality of the sub-group is high or, indeed, low. For example, in the above case the confidence interval surrounding the SMR of 69 for 'Professional workers, etc.' was 54–88, providing strong evidence that the mortality of these women was low.

Findings

Of the women aged 15–59 in 1971, 22 per cent were single; 73 per cent were married, of whom 47 per cent could be assigned an occupation, and the remainder were mainly housewives. Single women were heavily weighted towards the younger age groups; consequently (because death-rates are higher at older ages) they accounted for disproportionately few (10 per cent) of the deaths expected during 1976–81 to women aged 15–59, while married women accounted for 84 per cent.

We have intentionally omitted several residual groups which we know to have particularly high mortality as a result of the effects of health selection. Specifically, we have excluded women enumerated in institutions (a group which includes hospital patients), single women for whom we had no occupational information (these are mainly students but the mortality of the group was dominated by the permanently sick and disabled), and married women whose husbands could not be classified to an occupation (for example unemployed men who gave no details on their most recent job and those with inadequately described occupations).

Table 4.1 shows the mortality differences by own social class, housing tenure, and car access for single women, married women with an occupation, and married housewives. For married women differences by husband's social class are also given. The SMR is shown, along with the number of observed deaths and the 95 per cent Confidence Interval. The non-manual group encompasses social Classes I, II, and IIIN, while the manual group covers Social Classes IIIM, IV, and V. Although we have found it convenient to look at single and married women separately, comparisons between marital status categories are perfectly valid.

Table 4.1 Mortality 1976–81 of women aged 15–59 at death

| | Single women | | | Married women | | | | |
| | | | | With an occupation | | | Housewives | |
	SMR		95 % C.I.	SMR		95 % C.I.	SMR		95 % C.I.
Own social class									
Non-manual	84	(68)	65–105	79	(262)	69–89			
Manual	160	(62)	122–203	97	(310)	87–109			
Husband's social class									
Non-manual				72	(172)	62–84	71	(155)	60–83
Manual				96	(400)	87–106	121	(383)	109–134
Housing tenure									
Owner occupied	85	(48)	62–111	79	(269)	69–88	84	(258)	74–94
Private rented				93	(79)	73–115	111	(75)	87–138
Local authority rented	129	(82)	102–159	99	(223)	86–113	130	(203)	112–148
Cars in household									
Car(s)	80	(44)	57–105	83	(394)	75–92	83	(312)	74–92
No car	133	(86)	106–163	99	(177)	85–115	144	(224)	125–164
*All**	108	(130)	90–128	88	(572)	80–95	101	(538)	92–110

Source: OPCS Longitudinal Study (authors' analysis)

Notes: Figures in parentheses are numbers of observed deaths. Slight discrepancies occur in some totals due to non-response.

* As defined in this analysis i.e. excluding certain residual groups as described in the text.

© Crown Copyright

Single women, as a group, had raised mortality with an SMR of 108. Among married women, those with an occupation had the lowest mortality (SMR of 88), while housewives had an SMR of 101. These figures should not be interpreted to mean that being single is necessarily detrimental to women's health or, on the other hand, that being married and in work is beneficial. Health selection processes play an important role in producing these differences.

In the case of single women each characteristic divided the population into large groups with very different mortality levels. Low mortality was associated with non-manual occupations, owner-occupied housing, and having a car; conversely high mortality was associated with manual occupations, rented accommodation, and no car. For example, those in manual jobs had death-rates almost twice that of those in non-manual jobs; for housing tenure and access to cars, the 'disadvantaged' groups had death-rates about one and a half times that of the 'advantaged' groups. Among married women with an occupation there were also clear mortality differences in respect of each characteristic but they were much smaller than those for single women; the SMRs were all between 70 and 100. Differences by housing tenure and access to a car among housewives were very similar to those found among single women.

The household variables of housing tenure and access to cars are useful discriminators of mortality but they are not without problems. They relate to the household in which the woman was enumerated at census, and we can only speculate as to their meaning for the woman herself. Living in owner-occupied housing with a car provides an indicator of the overall material circumstances of the household, rather than telling us whether the woman herself owns the home, and/or has use of the car.

Although we have shown that each characteristic identifies high and low mortality groups, by using a combination of variables we have been able to take the analysis a stage further (Moser *et al.* 1988a). This has shown that further variations in mortality exist beyond those presented in Table 4.1, and that by cross-classifying women we can develop a more finely differentiated gradient. Table 4.2 summarizes the extent of the mortality differences and the characteristics which best describe the groups with particularly low and high SMRs.

For single women and housewives the range of mortality differences was extremely large (Table 4.2). In both cases the

Table 4.2 Summary of results

	Low mortality	High mortality	% of expected deaths covered by these 2 groups
1. Single women			
Characteristics	Non-manual	Manual	44%
	Car(s)	No car	
SMR (95% C.I.)	69 (47–98)	178 (131–236)	
Obs. (Exp.)dths.	30 (43.5)	48 (26.9)	
2. Married women			
a) *With an occupation*			
Characteristics	Non-manual	Manual	31%
	Husband non-manual	Husband manual	
	Owner occupier	Rented housing	
	Car(s)	No car	
SMR (95% C.I.)	70 (56–86)	113 (91–138)	
Obs. (Exp.) dths.	90 (129.3)	93 (82.0)	
b) *Housewives*			
Characteristics	Husband non-manual	Husband manual	44%
	Owner occupier	Rented housing	
	Car(s)	No car	
SMR (95% C.I.)	65 (53–79)	161 (135–188)	
Obs. (Exp.) dths.	104 (159.1)	147 (91.5)	

Source: OPCS Longitudinal Study (authors' analysis)
© Crown Copyright

differences were of a similar order of magnitude; the SMRs of the low mortality groups were just below 70, and those of the high mortality groups were 178 and 161 respectively. This means that for every 100 deaths in the low mortality group there were about 250 deaths in the high mortality group, after allowing for any differences in age structures. In the case of single women the main group with low mortality was that with the most favourable social circumstances (non-manual workers living in a household with a car). Conversely, the group which had none of these 'advantageous' characteristics had very high mortality. The number of deaths to single women were insufficient to allow a three-way classification so we have used occupation and car access as in this instance these variables were found to be the most useful discriminators of mortality. These two groups together represent a large and important component of the single population (accounting as they do for 44 per cent of the deaths expected among single women). Among housewives the low mortality group was those in owner-occupied housing, with a car, and whose husbands worked in a non-manual job, and the high mortality group those in rented housing, without a car, and whose husbands had a manual job.

In comparison with these exceptionally large differences in mortality, those found among married women with an occupation were small, ranging from an SMR of 70 in the low mortality group to 113 in the high mortality group. None the less, for every 100 deaths in the low mortality group there were about 160 deaths in the high mortality group. These differences are considerable given that they were found amongst a group of women who were 'selected' for good health at census: they were married; they were assigned an occupation, as were their husbands; and they lived in private households (rather than institutions or hospitals).

Table 4.2 shows very little difference between the SMRs of the low mortality groups. In contrast, among the high mortality groups, married women with an occupation do not appear to have the extreme disadvantage evident among single women or housewives. This may suggest a positive result of having two earners in the household.

The differences reported here are based on census measures which distinguish relative levels of advantage and disadvantage. Thus although possession of specific attributes described by these variables may directly affect mortality, it is primarily their value as effective descriptors of relative household wealth or poverty which lies behind the wide and consistent gradients found. It is important to note that all the characteristics we have described relate to 1971 and yet we are looking at mortality between 1976 and 1981 when these characteristics may well have altered, for example, a woman may have changed or left her job, she may have had a child, she may have become widowed or divorced. These changes in a woman's circumstances may have both immediate and delayed effects on her life and health. A further consideration is that the variables are clearly related, i.e., if you have a non-manual job you are more likely to own your home, have a car and, for married women, have a husband in a non-manual job. These are all advantageous characteristics in terms of mortality. Conversely manual jobs and rented accommodation without a car are, by comparison, disadvantageous characteristics.

By including household information we have been able to describe a woman's life circumstances more accurately than is possible using solely occupation-based measures. Information on occupation, housing tenure, and car access used in conjunction with marital status and economic activity has made it possible for us to develop a classification more appropriate to women's lives. By using a combination of characteristics we have demonstrated greater variation in mortality than that found using any one measure. For example, as Table 4.2 shows, the SMRs of married women with an occupation classified by a combination of characteristics range from 70 to 113, whereas using any one measure alone the range of SMRs is narrower (see Table 4.1). This is also the case for single women and married housewives. The differences we have focused on are those occurring among large groups of women; they do not simply represent exceptionally high death-rates among tiny groups.

We have made a preliminary analysis looking at other influences on women's lives (Moser et al. 1988b). Here we focus on married women with a dependent child. These are comparatively healthy women (young, married, with a child), and consequently we may expect their mortality to be fairly homogenous. However, this is far from the case as is shown in Table 4.3. There are large differences among those in paid employment. In particular among women working in non-manual jobs, those working full-time have much higher mortality than those working part-time. The high mortality of women in non-manual jobs working full-time might reflect the economic circumstances of the family, for example, an unemployed husband, rather than a direct effect of working full-time. Housewives married to men in manual jobs experienced death-rates over one and a half times as high as those married to men in non-manual jobs.

Overall, these results further confirm the need to consider other factors in conjunction with occupation, as even among married women in non-manual employment with dependent children there are large differences in mortality.

Table 4.3 Mortality 1976–81 of married women with a youngest child 0–16 years, by economic activity, own and husband's social class, and hours worked in 1971 (deaths at ages 15–59)

Own social class:	Non-manual	Manual	All
In paid employment			
Full-time	110 (85–139) (68)	89 (65–116) (47)	88 (78–99) (269)
Part-time	64 (48–82) (55)	95 (77–116) (99)	
Husband's social class:	*Non-manual*	*Manual*	*All*
Housewives	65 (52–80) (87)	107 (94–123) (217)	90 (30–101) (304)

SMR: (95% confidence interval)
(no. of observed deaths)

Source: OPCS Longitudinal Study (authors' analysis)
© Crown Copyright

Additional considerations

In addition to the influences on women's lives which we have considered here, there are other important aspects such as race or ethnic group, having elderly dependents, doing voluntary work, which we have been unable to incorporate in this analysis. This is because we are limited to the information collected at the 1971 Census and the size of the LS sample which does not allow for very detailed analyses when considering mortality in this age range.

The census economic activity categories are not clear-cut for many women and whether they (or whoever fills in the form on their behalf) describe themselves as in one, rather than another, category will depend on a variety of factors. For example, there is considerable overlap between 'housewife', 'unemployed', 'retired', and 'sick'. Factors which lead one woman to call herself a 'housewife' may well lead another to call herself 'unemployed'. In the present context the category 'housewife' poses a particular problem. Knowing only that a woman is a housewife tells us nothing about her social background. Indeed as we have seen there are big differences in the mortality of housewives according to whether they are married to men in non-manual or manual jobs, own or rent their homes, and whether they have a car.

The socio-economic categories identified here may be less relevant now than almost 20 years ago when this data was collected. Changes in women's employment patterns over recent years (such as an increase in part-time work), combined with demographic changes (such as increases in divorce and separation, the number of single women, one-parent families, and cohabitation) mean that husband's class has become even less appropriate as a sole measure of social classification for women.

Our knowledge about women's lives would be more complete if, in addition to asking about current employment, information was also sought about a woman's last job, including when it was. Details of a woman's current job provide no clues about the social circumstances of housewives, and could also be considered insufficient for women in employment whose current job may not reflect their skills, training, or potential. On the other hand it may be a good indicator of their resources. As Dex (1988) advocates, obtaining information on last job before childbearing may also be useful.

A composite social classification scheme for women has been developed by Barker and Roberts (1986) which incorporates several aspects of women's lives including occupation, the number of hours worked per week, and an assessment of their domestic responsibilities. In our work described here we have gone some way towards utilizing their approach, but in the future we hope to use the final version of their scheme for analysing women's mortality.

WHAT WE HAVE BEEN ABLE TO ACHIEVE AND WHY IT IS IMPORTANT

This analysis has shown how widely the mortality of women in England and Wales varies according to their social circumstances. This is further evidence (Townsend *et al.* 1988; Smith and Jacobson 1988) of the health inequalities which exist in our society. High mortality is associated with working in manual occupations, living in rented housing, and with no car in the household. In contrast low mortality is associated with non-manual occupations and living in owner-occupied housing with a car. Among housewives and single women the disadvantaged group experience death-rates two and a half times that of the advantaged group. Smaller differences are found among married women with an occupation. Among married women in employment differences are also found in the mortality of full- and part-time workers which relate to the woman's own social class; they are greater for those in non-manual than manual occupations.

We have shown that in order to accurately reflect the relationship between a woman's life circumstances and mortality it is necessary to use measures other than those based solely on occupation. By combining several simple indicators of socio-economic status, comparatively large groups may be constructed with greater differences in mortality than those that are apparent when using, for example, a finer differentiation of any one measure. Many of the relationships identified derive from simple empirical observations, such as the notion that the financial well-being and security associated with access to a car and home ownership are more commonly found among those in non-manual occupations. The value of this analysis has been to show how these inherent links may be exploited in the study of health differences.

Any study which hopes to group women using some form of social classification as a base could use the alternatives suggested here. The results presented in this chapter are for mortality from all causes of death, but other work has concentrated on specific causes of death. For example the relationship between smoking, lung cancer, and social circumstances has been examined using this approach (Pugh *et al.* 1989). Much of the information required for this alternative approach is already collected in surveys; hence we are not necessarily requesting additional data but simply a better and more imaginative use of existing material.

Any mortality studies which rely on occupational information from death registration are severely hampered by the incompleteness of recording of women's occupations. We would like to endorse strongly the suggestion made by Roman *et al.* (1985) that the Registrars' guidelines on the recording of women's occupations, last reviewed at the beginning of this century, are revised and made more appropriate to women's lives in the late twentieth century.

Unless the guidelines issued to registrars are modified, analyses relating women's occupations to disease will continue to suffer from the potential biases and difficulties associated with interpreting incomplete information.

(Roman *et al.* 1985: 196)

111

In terms of mortality, by pinpointing 'advantaged' and 'disadvantaged' groups of women in our society we get a better idea of how things could be, how they should be, and what we are working towards.

> ...the point of describing the stark class contrasts in illness and death rates in Britain today is not simply to chronicle a tragedy. The point about the gap between the health of the people at the top of society and that of the majority of people is that it is evidence that things do not have to be as they are. The health at present enjoyed by some people should be the right of all. . . . in a strange way knowledge of the class pattern of ill health can be an antidote to fatalism and resignation. It tells us our present suffering is not inevitable. . . . Better health is possible.
>
> (Mitchell 1984: 41)

ACKNOWLEDGEMENTS

1. We would like to thank Helen Roberts for her helpful advice and encouragement; also, members of the Social Statistics Research Unit, City University, especially Peter Goldblatt who has been very involved in the project, Michael Rosato for all his work on the computing, and Sharon Clarke for her clerical support.
2. Crown Copyright is reserved.
3. This work was supported by the Medical Research Council through grant No. G8203453.

Chapter Five

HYSTERECTOMY: A CHANGE OF TREND OR A CHANGE OF HEART?

PHILIP Y.K. TEO

There has been concern for some time, both within the medical profession and outside, about rising rates of hysterectomy. It is one of the most common major surgical operations in many countries (DHSS/OPCS 1985; Easterday *et al.* 1983; Roos 1984a; Pokras and Hufnagel 1988; Schacht and Pemberton 1985; Wijma *et al.* 1984) and, in the United States of America and Scotland, takes second place only to another controversial operation experienced only by women – caesarean section (Pokras and Hufnagel 1988; Scottish Health Statistics 1988).

In the United States of America the rate reached its highest in the mid-1970s with 670 operations per 100,000 female population and since then it has declined a little (Easterday *et al.* 1983; Pokras and Hufnagel 1988). In England and Wales the trend has been relatively stable over the last two decades after an initial increase in the mid-1960s (OPCS 1965–84). In England and Wales in 1983 over 60,000 hysterectomies were performed at a rate of 260 per 100,000 women per annum (DHSS/OPCS 1985) and more than 6,500 in Scotland at a rate of 249 per 100,000 women per annum (Scottish Health Statistics 1988). The lifetime risk of having a hysterectomy in the United States of America, based on the 1975 data, was 62 per cent (Perry 1976), i.e., more than half of American women would have lost their uteri in their lifetime. The risk in England and Wales is considerably lower at about 20 per cent (Alderson and Donnar 1978) and the Norwegian rates are half those of Britain (McPherson *et al.* 1982).

There are also large regional differences within countries. For example, in the United States of America, Walker and Jick (1979) found that for women under the age of 35 years, the hysterectomy rate in the south was three times higher than that in the north-east of the country. Loft *et al.* (1986) reported a sixfold variation in hysterectomy rates across Denmark. McPherson *et al.* (1981) demonstrated differences between geographical areas in England, Canada, and the USA.

It is, therefore, not surprising that hysterectomy is a controversial operation, and the controversy is further exacerbated by the finding that only a small proportion of hysterectomies are performed for life-threatening reasons and a large majority of the uteri removed were without demonstrable microscopic or macroscopic pathology. Miller, in 1946, drew attention to the fact that in 31 per cent of the cases he studied pathological examination revealed no evidence of disease. Less than 10 per cent of the hysterectomies were performed for diagnosed malignancies, the vast majority of the presenting symptoms being non-life-threatening conditions such as disorders of menstruation, fibroids, and genital prolapse (Amirikia and Evans 1979; Grant and Hussein 1984; Pokras and Hufnagel 1988).

Miller's (1946) provocative paper 'Hysterectomy: therapeutic necessity or surgical racket' strongly attacked the liberal use of hysterectomy. The paper was widely reported in the lay media and it began a public debate in North America. After Miller's paper, further studies have been carried out, not only by gynaecologists, but also by the American truck drivers' union, by insurance companies, and, in 1974, by the US Congress (Open University 1985).

While the medical profession's concern about the escalating rates is exemplified in the following self-regulation, the same might be used as evidence of an inappropriately high startingpoint, which called for regulation. In the Province of Saskatchewan, Canada, Dyck *et al.* (1977) reported a surveillance system to monitor hysterectomies. They found that the number of hysterectomies performed dropped dramatically after a medical committee started monitoring the reasons for which the operations were performed. Mandatory second-opinion programmes have also led to a decrease in the rate at which discretionary surgery is performed (Grafe *et al.* 1978).

In addition to the debate about the indication for hysterectomy, there has been some argument about the 'usefulness' of the uterus. Wright (1969) claimed in an editorial, for instance, that 'the uterus has but one function: reproduction. After the last planned pregnancy, the uterus becomes a useless, bleeding, symptom-producing, potentially cancer-bearing organ and should be removed' (p. 561). Leaving to one side this radical approach, it is worthwhile examining the risks of the prophylactic hysterectomy advocated.

Richards (1973, 1974) demonstrated that depression requiring treatment was common after hysterectomy and coined the term 'post-hysterectomy syndrome'. He also suggested a possible endocrine function of the uterus. However, a prospective study by Gath *et al.* (1982) concluded that although the operation may have affected some women badly, in the majority of cases positive psychological improvements were recorded.

Another association which has been explored is that between hysterectomy and cardio-vascular disease. A pre-menopausal simple hysterectomy was found to be associated with a threefold increase in the subsequent incidence and prevalence of coronary heart disease during the remaining pre-menopausal years. In the ten-year follow-up there was a 4 per cent probability of coronary heart disease and 0.04 per cent of dying from it (Centrewall 1981). The mechanism of the association is not clear but it was not due to differences in oestrogen use, cigarette smoking, or relative weight gain. This association provides a new lead in coronary disease research and a further rebuttal to Wright's argument.

From a health economics perspective, Bunker *et al.* (1977) calculated that elective hysterectomy and oophorectomy in a 40-year-old healthy woman would result in a net gain in life expectancy of fourteen days; however, if hysterectomy alone is performed leaving the ovaries intact (i.e. a potential risk of ovarian cancer) the estimated increase in life expectancy is reduced to four days. Sandberg *et al.* (1983), using newer data, calculated the comparable figures as 0.43 and 0.18 years. The later study concluded that gains in life expectancy and quality of life can be expected when women aged 30–60 undergo hysterectomy for benign neoplasm, disorders of menstruation, acquired abnormal anatomy (such as genital prolapse), cervical disease, or endometriosis, due primarily to prevention of reproductive tract cancers, which outweigh the impact of operative mortality. But women who have relatively high operative risk or low expected cancer risk will be likely to suffer losses in life expectancy.

Burnham, in 1853, performed the first 'successful' hysterectomy. Only three of the fifteen patients survived. While Burnham lost 80 per cent of his patients, the current mortality rate for hysterectomy is 0.02 per cent (Open University 1985). As the safety of the operation improved, the indications for hysterectomy liberalized to the extent of routine prophylactic removal of uterus advocated by Wright in 1969.

During the period between Burnham and Wright, hysterectomy has, therefore, moved from being an operation of the last resort to something that is urged, by some gynaecologists, for the removal of the symptomless uterus.

Hysterectomy is an operation which has aroused considerable interest both from within and outside the medical profession because of its high rate of use and the apparent liberal indications for the operation. The hysterectomy debate has resulted in numerous studies, so it is surprising that little work has been done on the epidemiology of hysterectomy in Scotland. With the exception of the study by Grant and Hussein (1984), which is an audit of abdominal hysterectomy over a period of ten years in a Scottish district hospital, there is no other study of hysterectomy in Scotland in the literature. This is especially interesting because the Scottish rate is rising while other western countries are experiencing a downward or stable trend.

THE SCOTTISH STUDY

This study is a retrospective analysis made on the basis of routinely collected health information, the Scottish Morbidity Record 1 (SMR1). The SMR1 record relates to all patients discharged from non-psychiatric, non-obstetric wards in Scottish Health Service hospitals.

The scheme is episode-based and records the discharge from a speciality, which is defined by the speciality of the consultant in charge of the patient. A discharge record is therefore raised when a patient changes consultant or is transferred to another hospital. The number of records increased from 436,545 in 1961 to over three-quarters of a million records 24 years later in 1985. The SMR1 is unique, being a population-based data set with a high degree of completeness and validity.

The data in this chapter are based on the SMR1 record of

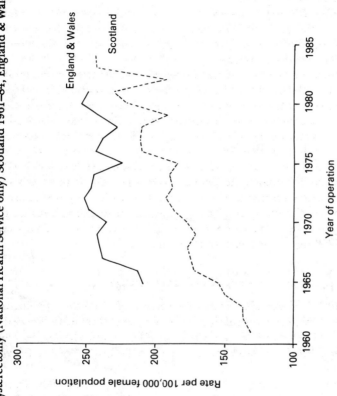

Figure 5.1 Hysterectomy (National Health Service only) Scotland 1961–84, England & Wales 1965–81

Sources: SMR1 & HIPE (author's analysis)

121,147 hysterectomies performed in the Scottish Health Service hospitals during the period 1961 to 1984.

FINDINGS

General trend over time

The time trends of hysterectomy in Scotland from 1961 to 1984, and England and Wales for 1965 to 1981, are shown in Figure 5.1. It should be noted that hysterectomies performed outside the National Health Service are not included. The NHS rate for England and Wales was fairly stable over that period while the Scottish trend, starting from a lower rate in the 1960s, has increased steadily and is catching up with England and Wales. The Scottish rate has almost doubled in that 24-year period. The 'dips' in 1975, 1979, and 1982 were the years of major union action which disrupted the health service. Using the 1980 rates for comparison, the Scottish rate was 15 per cent less than that of England and Wales and was two and a half times less than the rates in the USA.

Time trends by age groups

In Figure 5.2 the annual rate of hysterectomy is divided into six broad age groups. The group aged 0 to 24 years is excluded from the analysis because of the negligible number of hysterectomies performed below the age of 24 years. The two groups showing the steepest increase are those aged 35–44 and 45–54 years. The youngest group, 25–34 years, also shows an upward trend but not as striking as that for the other two groups. Over the age of 55 years the operative rate shows little change over the 24-year period. It is interesting to note the 'dips' in 1975, 1979, and 1982. As pointed out earlier, these were the years of major union disputes, and the drop in the number of operations affected the different age groups with different degrees of severity. The dips are deepest in the 35–44 age group.

What is the lifetime risk of hysterectomy?

Another way of presenting the age-specific data is to calculate the cumulative probability of hysterectomy based on the method of

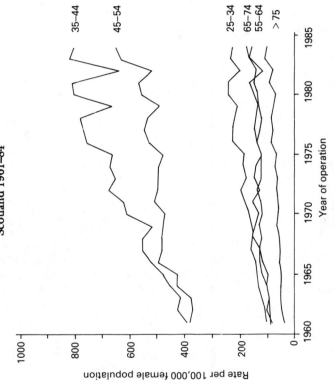

Figure 5.2 Hysterectomy by age groups,
Scotland 1961–84

Source: SMR1 (author's analysis)

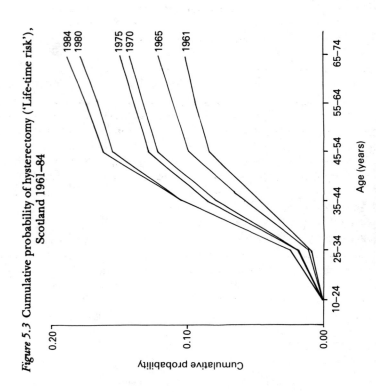

Figure 5.3 Cumulative probability of hysterectomy ('Life-time risk'), Scotland 1961–84

Source: SMR1 (author's analysis)

Bunker *et al.* (1977). It is possible to estimate the cumulative probability that a woman would undergo hysterectomy in Scotland were she to be subjected throughout life to the age-specific hysterectomy rate for a specific year. Figure 5.3 shows the cumulative probability for selected years.

In 1961, in Scotland, the risk of a woman having a hysterectomy by the age of 74 years was 10 per cent. This risk has increased progressively over the years, as indicated by the shifting of the successive curves towards the left, so that by 1984 the risk was almost 19 per cent. The risk in England and Wales also shows a similar trend, although the risk of 1975 dropped below that of 1970; the risk in England in 1984 was 21 per cent. In the United States of America the risk was 62 per cent (Perry 1976) when the rate of hysterectomy was at its highest; the current American rate is around 37 per cent (Pokras and Hufnagel 1988).

Why do women have hysterectomies?

The analysis of the diagnostic reasons for hysterectomy was carried out using eleven major categories, by regrouping the International Classification of Diseases (ICD) codings. Table 5.1 is a summary of the proportion in each category for 1984.

Table 5.1 Diagnostic categories for hysterectomy, Scotland, 1984

	Number	*Percentage*
Menstrual disorders	2,271	34.9
Fibroids	1,317	20.2
Genital prolapse	605	9.3
Malignant neoplasms	525	8.1
Pelvic inflammatory disease	108	1.7
Carcinoma *in situ* (cervix)	88	1.4
Postmenopausal bleeding	87	1.3
Benign neoplasms *	77	1.2
Others	1,436	22.0
Total	6,514	100.1

Source: SMR1 (Scottish Morbidity Records 1, 1984) (author's analysis)
Note: * fibroids excluded.

Table 5.1 shows that the biggest category of indication for hysterectomy is menstrual disorders, which accounted for almost 35 per cent of the hysterectomies performed in the Scottish Health Service in 1984. The first three categories represent over two-thirds of the cases. Malignant neoplasms were the indication for 8.1 per cent of the cases.

How have diagnostic reasons for hysterectomy changed over time?

The time trends of a selected diagnostic group are shown in Figure 5.4. In the interest of continuity carcinoma *in situ* of the cervix and post-menopausal bleeding are excluded because these new codes were not introduced into SMR1 until 1968; pelvic inflammatory disease is excluded because coding changes mean that one would not be comparing strictly equivalent groups. The 'others' group is also excluded for clarity of presentation and because of its heterogeneity. The selected groups represent more than 70 per cent of all cases of hysterectomy performed from 1961–84.

Over the period studied menstrual disorders have always been the commonest diagnostic category; at around 1970 the rate rises sharply with a widening gap between this category and other groups. The trends for the other groups are relatively stable with the exception of benign neoplasms which shows a slight decline in recent years.

For a closer look at the menstrual disorders, the trends for three selected age groups are presented in Figure 5.5. The picture here is very similar to Figure 5.2 for the overall rates for hysterectomies. The group with the steepest increase is the 35–44 age group and, as in Figure 5.3, the rate again increases sharply at around 1970 which is clearly shown for the age group 35–44 years, where the 1984 rate is 60 per cent greater than that for 1970.

Deaths from hysterectomy

The number of cases which, on discharge from the hospital, were coded as dead was used as a figure for deaths directly or indirectly due to hysterectomy; though other definitions might have been used. Buck *et al.* (1988), for instance, look at perioperative mortality in terms of death within 30 days of an operation, but these data are not routinely available.

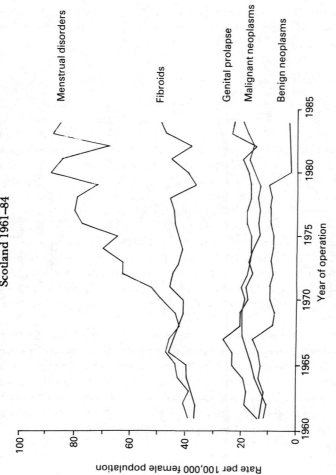

Figure 5.4 Hysterectomy by selected diagnostic categories,
Scotland 1961–84

Source: SMR1 (author's analysis)

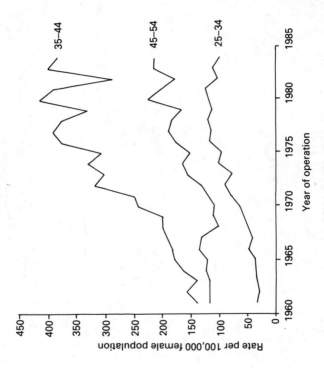

Figure 5.5 Hysterectomy for menstrual disorders by selected age groups, Scotland 1961–84

Source: SMR1 (author's analysis)

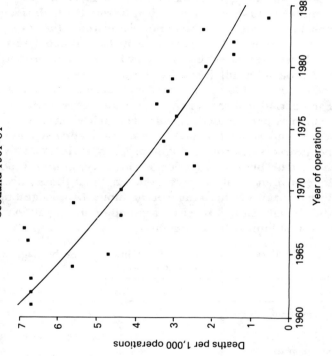

Figure 5.6 'Operative' mortality from hysterectomy, Scotland 1961–84

Source: SMR1 (author's analysis)

During the period 1961–84 the total number of deaths associated with hysterectomy was 447 out of the total of 121,147 hysterectomies performed, which gave a gross operative mortality of 3.7 per 1,000 operations. The rate of operative mortality is presented in Figure 5.6 which shows a reassuring downward trend. In 1961 the mortality rate was 6.7 per 1,000 hysterectomies and by 1984 the mortality rate was 0.6 per 1,000 hysterectomies, which represents more than an elevenfold improvement in the mortality associated with the operation. In 1984 the mortality rate of 0.06 per cent was entirely due to four deaths from the high risk group of malignancies and there were no deaths from other categories. In other words, with the exception of malignant neoplasms, Scotland achieved zero operative mortality in 1984. The proportional contribution of death from the diagnostic categories over the period of 1961 to 1984 is presented in Table 5.2, which shows that over the period malignant neoplasm is the largest contributor of more than 44 per cent of the deaths. This in itself may be cause for concern, and some of these operations may well have been desperate measures which might properly and humanely have been avoided. Buck *et al.* (1988), for instance, in their report on perioperative mortality, express concern about those operations performed at an advanced stage of carcinomatosis, suggesting that careful thought should be given to whether an operation should be performed under these circumstances.

Table 5.2 Total deaths associated with hysterectomy by diagnostic categories – Scotland 1961–84

	Number	*Percentage*
Malignant neoplasms	198	44.3
Fibroids	38	8.5
Prolapse (genital)	37	8.3
Benign neoplasms	22	4.9
Menstrual disorders	19	4.3
Postmenopausal bleeding	10	2.2
Abd and GI tract related	5	1.1
Pelvic inflammatory disease	4	0.9
Carcinoma *in situ* (cervix)	1	0.2
Congenital abnormality	1	0.2
Others	112	25.1
Total	447	100

Source: SMR1 (Scottish Morbidity Records 1, 1961–84) (author's analysis)

Cross-boundary flow of hysterectomy

In Scotland the delivery of health services is divided into fifteen geographical areas (health boards), each with its own catchment population. The division is, however, a flexible one which allows for patients from one catchment area to be treated elsewhere. This type of movement of patients between health boards is called cross-boundary flow. There are considerable movements between health boards with the largest 'importer' showing a net gain of 25 per cent of its cases and the smaller health boards 'exporting' almost all their cases to other boards. Because of the cross-boundary flow, it is not possible to have an acceptable denominator for analysis of regional differences within Scotland. One of the solutions is to divide the Scottish mainland health boards into 'East' and 'West' regions. By doing so the net flow of cases between the 'East HBs' and 'West HBs' was negligible. Ninety-two, or 0.65 per cent, of cases from the 'East HBs' were operated on by the 'West HBs' and 69, or 0.44 per cent, cases from the 'West' were treated in the 'East'. Hence it is possible to compare the two regions. While a comparison across regions may, at first sight, appear parochial to the non-Scottish reader, this has important implications in understanding denominator problems, as discussed later. These problems are relevant to anyone who might be using small area statistics to look at regional differences in health services utilization.

Regional differences

During the period 1980–4 the Eastern health boards performed more hysterectomies than the West; the age standardized rate for the East is about 10 per cent higher. Surprisingly, given the overall trends shown in Figure 5.5, the differences are in the older age groups, i.e. over the age of 45 years.

Table 5.3 shows the differences between the East and West for selected diagnostic categories. Apart from two relatively small groups – pelvic inflammatory disease and carcinoma *in situ* of the cervix – the East performed more operations than the West. There are large differences in the number of hysterectomies performed for genital prolapse and benign neoplasms. It is especially interesting to note the 47 per cent difference for operations performed for malignant neoplasms.

127

Table 5.3 Hysterectomy rates (NHS) by selected diagnostic categories 'Eastern' and 'Western' Scottish Health Boards, 1980–84

	* *Eastern* H.Bs	* *Western* H.Bs	*Ratio* East:West	*p*
Menstrual disorders	81.6	65.4	1.25	0.0001
Fibroids	46.9	40.9	1.15	0.0001
Genital prolapse	25.6	14.4	1.78	0.0001
Malignant neoplasms	20.9	14.2	1.47	0.0001
Benign neoplasms	3.5	1.9	1.84	0.0001
Pelvic inflammatory disease	2.7	3.5	0.77	0.01
Carcinoma *in situ* (cervix)	2.2	6.2	0.35	0.0001

Source: SMR1 (Scottish Morbidity Records 1, 1980–84) (author's analysis)
Note: * rate per 100,000 female population.

Relationship of time trends of hysterectomy and health service variables

Number of consultant gynaecologists

The number of consultant gynaecologists and the rate of operation per consultant from 1961 to 1984 is given in Figures 5.7 and 5.8. The establishment of consultant gynaecologists expanded rapidly from the early 1960s and reached a relatively stable state in the early 1970s, by which time the number of posts for consultant gynaecologists was almost one and a half times that of 1960. Interestingly, the rate of hysterectomy per consultant per year accelerated at around the 1970s as shown in Figure 5.8. The correlation of the hysterectomy rate by number of consultant gynaecologists for the period 1961–84 using the Spearman rank correlation (r) is 0.95 which is highly significant. In essence this means that the more gynaecologists there are, the more operations there are. This finding will be discussed further below.

Waiting time, duration of stay and beds

The mean time on the waiting list in days and the mean duration of stay in days in hospital for hysterectomy is shown in Figure 5.9. There is a general decrease in the duration of stay from an average of 19 days in 1961 to 11.5 days in 1984; there is a general increase in the mean waiting time from 34.3 days in 1961 to 58.2 days in 1984.

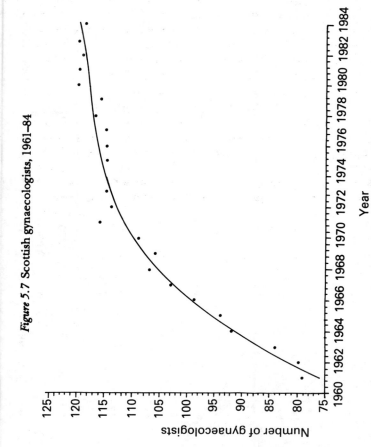

Figure 5.7 Scottish gynaecologists, 1961–84

Source: Scottish Health Statistics 1961–84

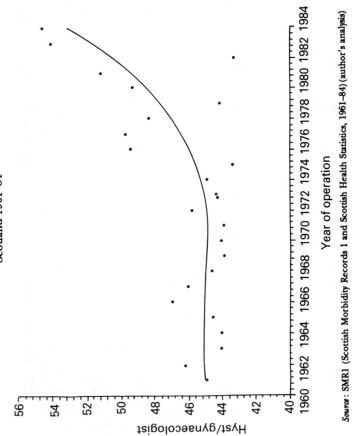

Figure 5.8 Hysterectomy per gynaecologist, Scotland 1961–84

Year of operation

Hyst/gynaecologist

Source: SMR1 (Scottish Morbidity Records 1 and Scottish Health Statistics, 1961–84) (author's analysis)

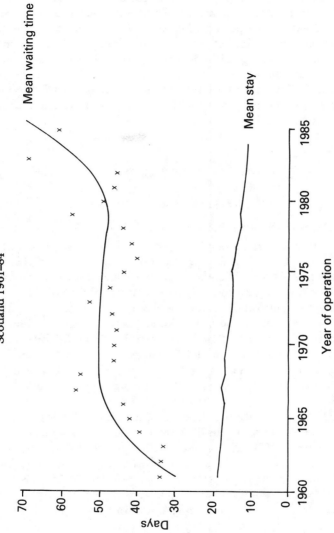

Figure 5.9 Mean waiting time and post-operative stay (days) for hysterectomy, Scotland 1961–84

Source: SMR1 (Scottish Morbidity Records 1 and Scottish Health Statistics, 1961–84) (author's analysis)

The correlation of the hysterectomy rate with waiting time, duration of stay, and available staffed gynaecological beds was calculated for the period 1970 to 1984 and indicated a significant negative correlation between the hysterectomy rate and number of staffed gynaecological beds, and between the hysterectomy rate and mean duration of stay for the period 1970–84. What this means is that more hysterectomies were being performed with a decreasing number of available beds and a shorter length of stay after the operation.

DISCUSSION

Materials and methods of the study

Data source: Scottish Morbidity Record 1

This study is a retrospective analysis of routinely collected health statistics, SMR1. It is a unique national data set which covers the whole population of Scotland; however, it excludes operations performed outside National Health Service hospitals. There is no figure available on the extent of private hysterectomies performed in Scotland. In England and Wales, private hysterectomies were estimated to be more than 20 per cent in 1984 (Nicholl *et al* 1984) with considerable regional differences. In Scotland, private hysterectomies are estimated to be about 5 per cent, based on an informal audit of the workload of a group of gynaecologists (Webb 1986).

The next question is how complete is SMR1? While it is not possible to ascertain this directly, it is possible to check indirectly using the ISD(S)1 (Information and Statistical Division) which is another set of hospital activity statistics concerned with the bed utilization within Scottish hospitals. It is independent of SMR1 and provides information about bed usage. In-patient statistics include data such as bed complement, waiting list, staffed bed days, occupied beds, and discharges. In repeated completeness checks performed by the Information and Statistical Division (ISD) by comparison of SMR1 returns with ISD(S)1 returns the SMR1 has been found to be well over 96 per cent complete.

Validity of SMR1

The validity of SMR1 has two aspects: first, there is the transcription and coding accuracy of SMR1 and, second, the validity of SMR1 data in terms of factual information in the medical case notes.

There are two major transcription and coding validity studies. The first was by Lockwood (1971), in which a 0.5 per cent sample of discharges from 38 major hospitals in Scotland was studied over a three-month period in 1969. The second study by Smith (1981) was based on a 1 per cent sample of discharges from the major hospitals in the Greater Glasgow Health Board for the year 1981. The overall validity of all the items recorded was 96.7 per cent for the first study and 95.1 per cent for the second. There were, however, considerable variations of error rates for specific items of SMR1 which range from less than 1 per cent for patient's name and sex to more than 30 per cent for secondary diagnoses. The major errors were found to be largely due to omissions in the information rather than transcription and coding mistakes. The error rates for the items used in this study are summarized in Table 5.4. With the exception of the higher error rate for waiting time of the earlier study, all other items used in this study have an accuracy of over 90 per cent. It was not possible to analyse the data by social class because of the high error of almost 20 per cent. The social class data is no longer routinely collected for SMR1.

Table 5.4 Selected items of error rates for SMR1 1971 and 1981

	Lockwood's study (1971) No. of errors (%)		Smith's study (1981) No. of errors (%)	
Date of birth	94	(3.7)	46	(3.6)
Waiting list date	159	(14.8)	40	(7.6)
Admission date	42	(1.7)	24	(1.9)
Discharge date	90	(3.6)	23	(1.9)
Discharge code	15	(0.6)	9	(0.7)
Diagnostic data (1st)	157	(6.3)	104	(8.3)
Main operation	123	(10.3)	59	(9.3)
Post code	131	(5.2)	59	(4.9)

Source: Adapted from Lockwood (1971) and Smith (1981)

Although the geographical bases of the two validation studies were different they indicated stability of error rates between the two studies which is an important consideration for analysis over a long duration.

In addition to the transcription and coding accuracy of SMR1, Patel *et al.* (1976) demonstrated the poor concurrent validity of SMR1 diagnostic data and factual information due to inaccurate extraction of information. Patel *et al.* found in 1976 that there was 19 per cent underestimation of self-poisoning and a 17 per cent error rate in the main diagnosis for myocardial infarction. The study was, however, based on one hospital, which may not be representative, and the validity checks were on two clinical entities where the scope for multiple diagnostic labelling was considerable. Smith's study confirms the poor accuracy of diagnostic data indicated by Patel but there are large variations between specialities – for gynaecology the diagnostic error rate was 5.7 per cent with an overall error rate of 3.7 per cent. It is thus reasonable to accept that the SMR1 data set for the speciality of gynaecology is complete and has acceptable validity for the purpose of this study.

Denominator problems

The denominator is based on the population at risk in the calculation of a rate or ratio, for example, hysterectomies per 100,000 women. This is fundamental to epidemiological studies as it allows the characteristics of one population to be compared with another. The denominator must, therefore, be valid and appropriate. Because of cross-boundary flow of cases of hysterectomy between health boards, a problem arises when examining the differences between health boards. We need to distinguish between the treatment catchment population and the resident population. The treatment population can be larger or smaller than the resident population depending on whether the health board is a net importer or exporter of cases. Studies of regional differences tend to ignore this problem and use the resident population as the denominator. This is, of course, invalid. Using the resident population as the denominator in a net 'importing' health board will, in effect, exaggerate the workload of the health board; the net gained cases inflate the numerator but not the denominator and, conversely, underestimate the workload of a net 'exporting' health board.

The two solutions to the above problem were to compare two geographical areas and the estimated catchment population. By dividing Scotland into East and West the cross-boundary bias became negligible. The denominator used for East and West comparison was the aggregated resident female population for the two groups of health boards over the period 1980 to 1984. Similarly, the numerator was the aggregated cases of hysterectomies performed over the same period. It was necessary to aggregate the five-year data so as to overcome the fluctuation created by industrial action over the period.

The catchment population for gynaecology patients was provided by the Information and Statistical Division. It is based on the proportionate flow method (Pinder 1982) which is a relatively straightforward method of estimating catchment population provided the data for cross-boundary flow is available. Even without full cross-boundary flow data, Pinder demonstrated that good estimates of catchment populations can be made with relatively small samples of cases from different health districts. If the catchment population can be calculated or estimated with relative ease and with good accuracy, then the improper use of the resident population as the denominator when there is significant cross-boundary flow should be discouraged.

Trends over time

It is interesting to observe the narrowing gap in the rate of hysterectomy between Scotland, England, and Wales, although the figure for England and Wales may be confounded by hysterectomies performed outside the NHS (Coulter et al. 1988). Why should there be such differences between countries operating similar health care systems? What are the factors behind the increasing rate in Scotland? While it is not possible to answer the first question with this study it is possible to demonstrate the major components behind the increase in Scotland.

The rise has been largely due to the steady increase in the rate of hysterectomies performed for menstrual disorders in the age group 35–44 years. This observation is well-established but has not been so clearly demonstrated by other studies (Traub *et al.* 1980; Grant and Hussein 1984; Wijma *et al.* 1984).

It is intriguing to note that the rate of increase in hysterectomy appeared during the 1970s, a time when the number of consultant gynaecologists reached its stable level, and at a time when the number of available staffed gynaecology beds was on the decrease. This paradoxical observation can be explained by the increase in the 'efficiency' of gynaecologists, demonstrated by their rate of operation for hysterectomy accelerating during the 1970s while the duration of stay for the operation was reduced. The increase in efficiency, no doubt, is partly due to the changes in the case-mix of hysterectomy; that is, the differences in the characteristics of the population for the operation. Many of those having the operation are now from the younger and fitter group and with relatively straightforward, less time-consuming hysterectomies performed for menstrual disorders.

The observed increased use of surgical treatment for menstrual disorders is puzzling particularly because, since the early 1970s, the physiology of menstruation has been better understood along with the roles of hormonal control and the discovery of the function of prostaglandins. This was a period when there were increasing numbers of pharmacologically distinct agents available for the conservative treatment of menstrual disorders (Nobel 1985). It is interesting to note that Miller (1946) foresaw that 'non-surgical control of this troublesome symptom (endocrinal uterine bleeding) appears to be more than just a pipe-dream' (p. 805). Although we now have an array of medical remedies surgical treatment continues to dominate the management of menstrual disorders.

The cumulative probability of hysterectomy during a woman's lifetime in Scotland is around 19 per cent. The calculation is based on the assumption that the same hysterectomy rate is applied over the lifetime of the female cohort. However, in view of the increasing trend, the Scottish figure is likely to be an under-estimation. The American lifetime risk at present is 37 per cent (Pokras and Hufnagel 1988) and it is difficult to conceive that more than one-third of American women need a hysterectomy.

It will be of great interest to watch the Scottish trend over the next few years: is it going to slow down and stabilize, as it should be, or will it continue on its accelerating course heading for the higher American rate?

The reasons for hysterectomy

Menstrual disorders is the largest diagnostic category for hysterectomy accounting for almost 35 per cent of cases. The malignant neoplasms group accounted for about 8 per cent of all cases. The relative proportions of the diagnostic indications correspond roughly with other studies (Amirikia and Evans 1979; Grant and Hussein 1984). Miller's paper (1946), based on this type of analysis, strongly attacked the liberal use of hysterectomy. In one-third of the cases of his analysis of 246 hysterectomies, he found no evidence of pathology. Following this paper, a major study was performed (Doyle 1953) in which the conclusion was that 21.5 per cent of the cases were regarded as unnecessary hysterectomies; Dyck et al. (1977) reached similar conclusions.

What is an unnecessary operation? It is almost impossible to measure with any degree of certainty to what extent unnecessary surgery is carried out. Rutkow (1982) pointed out that any evaluation is handicapped by the lack of a generally accepted definition of unnecessary surgery due to disagreement on the indication for many operations. In many instances, unnecessary hysterectomy is equated with the removal of a 'normal' uterus when examined macroscopically and microscopically. With medical knowledge now extended beyond the microscopic level to subcellular and molecular level, should the traditional pathological examination still be regarded as the gold standard for normality? And should the removal of apparently normal organs for symptomatic relief be regarded as unnecessary? This is a difficult question to answer because it is outside the normal boundary of medical decision-making. Psychosocial and ethical considerations are involved, and who should decide?

The necessity for hysterectomy should not be judged simply in terms of 'hard' measures of physical morbidity and mortality; it must be extended to fulfil the WHO definition of health, i.e. complete physical, mental, and social well-being. That is, women's own experiences of having hysterectomies should be taken into account and women must be given the opportunity to be fully involved in the decision-making process (Coulter et al. 1988).

Deaths from hysterectomy

The number of cases which on discharge from the hospital were coded as dead was assumed to be the figure for deaths directly or indirectly due to hysterectomy. It is, therefore, not strictly operative mortality but deaths associated with hysterectomy. A small number of deaths may not have been included here if the critically ill patient was being transferred from a different speciality within the same hospital and also cases readmitted after a recent hysterectomy. Cases dying soon after discharge would also be missed. These numbers are likely to be small in the majority of operations performed for non-malignant reasons.

The overall downward trend of the mortality associated with hysterectomy over the study is reassuring. The safety of the operation is clearly related to the age of the patient and the diagnostic indication. Forty-four per cent of the deaths were due to 8 per cent of the total cases performed for malignant neoplasms. The downward trend is, therefore, exaggerated by the greater selection of younger and fitter patients for uncomplicated operations. It is, however, reasonably demonstrated that the decrease is happening within all diagnostic groups especially the malignant neoplasms. The drop in the last group may also be due to selection bias. Since it is now possible to 'stage' the malignancy without laparotomy by the use of laparoscopy and computer assisted scanners, it may be that 'good and early' cases are selected for operative treatment while the advanced cases are treated by radiotherapy and chemotherapy.

The mortality data of this study is a major series. There are other major studies in North America (Wingo *et al.* 1985). The Scottish overall mortality rate over the whole study period was 3.7 per 1,000 operations, which is high compared with the two American series of 1.2 and 1.5 per 1,000 operations. This may, however, be an unfair comparison as the American studies are based on more recent data. The mortality figure for Scotland from 1980 to 1984 was, in fact, 1.6 per 1,000 operations which is comparable to the American figures. But the comparison of the crude rate is of little use – as already discussed it very much depends on the case-mix of the series, that is, how many of the women were at serious risk from age or illness to begin with?

Regional differences

It is interesting to note the age standardized rate of hysterectomy in the East is higher than in the West by a magnitude of about 10 per cent and yet the East over the same duration had fewer gynaecologists – 4.0 per 100,000 female population compared with 4.3 per 100,000 female population in the West. The East also had fewer staffed gynaecology beds (43.3 per 100,000 female population for the East and 74.6 per 100,000 female population for the West). This observation apparently contradicts the notion that the surgical work-load is in direct proportion to the availability of surgical resources, particularly manpower (Lewis 1969; Bunker 1970; Wennberg and Gittelsohn 1973; McPherson *et al.* 1981).

The East and West comparison also indicates a different pattern of case-mix. The East performed more hysterectomies in the older age groups, especially the over-75 age group, than the West. The mix of diagnostic indication is also very different between the two regions. In the East there were operations on 47 per cent more malignant neoplasms and 78 per cent more pelvic floor repairs. The difference may simply reflect different clinical thinking and practice, it may represent a difference in morbidity between the two regions or it may reflect the fact that the 'East' had more 'teaching' consultants. Unfortunately, it is not possible to answer these questions without a detailed study of the prevalence of gynaecological problems and a survey of the clinical practice of the consultants from both sides.

Waiting time and length of stay

The overall mean waiting time for hysterectomy has increased from 34 to 58 days over the 24-year study period, which is an increase of 70 per cent. The increase, when broken down for diagnostic indications, appears to come from menstrual disorders and fibroids; the mean waiting time for other diagnoses is relatively stable. This could be interpreted as an increase in demand or need or an increased inclination of surgeons to operate in these two categories.

The overall length of stay for hysterectomy fell from 19 to 11.5 days over the study period, which is a fall of 40 per cent; the fall for the main diagnostic groups is similar. This fall reflects mainly the change in medical thinking about post-operative care, especially early mobilization. The shortened length of stay, no doubt, also helps to improve the 'efficiency' of gynaecologists.

Using the mean length of stay and the percentage occupancy figure, it is possible to calculate the proportion of gynaecology beds 'consumed' by hysterectomy. In 1975, hysterectomy accounted for about 33 per cent of total occupied gynaecology beds; by 1984 this figure had increased to 45 per cent. Hysterectomy, therefore, is the major activity in the gynaecology wards, with almost half of the resources geared towards it. Therefore, in addition to other controversial issues surrounding hysterectomy, it is a high consumer of gynaecological service resources. It is estimated that each hysterectomy costs the NHS about £1000 (Coulter *et al.* 1988) which represents a total value of over £6.5 million in 1984 in Scotland.

Correlation analysis

The correlation of the hysterectomy rate by the number of consultant gynaecologists for 1961 to 1984 produced a highly significant relationship with r=0.95. What is the significance of this?

First of all, it is important to stress that association does not necessarily mean causation. In the above two situations it is necessary to examine the variables more closely. In the correlation, the consultants are assumed to be a collection of homogeneous variables – which in practice is far from true. Consultant gynaecologists in Scotland are also obstetricians – the split of their time between the two specialities is not always an equal division. In correlation analysis it would have been more valid to correlate the rate of hysterectomy with the number of gynaecological sessions, but data for this was not available.

For the dependent variable, hysterectomy rate, the analysis assumes all the hysterectomies are the same without the consideration of the diagnostic reason for which the operation is indicated. Clinical practice and thinking do change over time and vary in different places. Morbidity patterns may change over time and there may be regional variations in gynaecological morbidity.

It is apparent that the correlation analysis of the overall hysterectomy rate by the number of consultant gynaecologists is of limited value and should be interpreted with caution. With these shortcomings in mind, the relationship of the hysterectomy rate to staffing levels is inconclusive. If the East and West comparison is taken into account, i.e. the East performed more hysterectomies with fewer gynaecologists, the balance of evidence would appear to contradict the general observation of the apparent relationship of surgical staffing level and surgical output. It must be stressed, however, that there may be differences in the types of consultants in the two regions; three of the four teaching boards are in the East, but the single largest teaching board is in the West.

EXPLANATIONS

In this final section of discussion the possible explanations for the changes over time and regional differences in hysterectomy will be explored with special reference to the findings reported in this chapter.

McPherson *et al.* (1981) listed the possible sources of variations in rates of surgery based on geographical areas, which are as listed below:

1 age and sex composition
2 age-specific disease incidence
3 random variation with time and place
4 availability, e.g. a manpower
                  b hospital bed provision
                  c funding
                  d waiting lists
                  e methods of payment
5 clinical judgement
6 variation in patient demand or expectation
7 rate of organ removal in previous years
8 prevailing custom
9 systematic omissions of operations, e.g. private surgery, day cases
10 differences in coding procedures
11 inaccuracies in information sources

It is a comprehensive list. Although it is set out for a discussion of regional difference, it is also valid for analysis of change over time. The list is, however, slightly too detailed for our purposes. In this discussion the list is regrouped into five main factors, namely:

1 morbidity factors
2 resource/supply factors
3 clinician characteristics
4 patient characteristics
5 artefacts

Morbidity factors

It is possible that changes over time and regional differences could simply be a matter of geographical differences in morbidity rates and changes in the morbidity pattern over time. In most investigations this is seen as unlikely, and it is argued that relative morbidity differences could not account for these large variations (Coulter and McPherson 1986). But this assumption can be challenged. It is possible that changes in morbidity have altered the indications for hysterectomy. There are no reliable data on the prevalence of gynaecological morbidity in the population; it is, therefore, impossible to refute or prove the assumption. But one can at least speculate that changes in reproductive patterns and the use of oral contraception could influence menstrual disorders over the time of the study period.

This chapter clearly demonstrates the changing pattern of diagnostic indications for hysterectomy. Since the 1970s there has been a large relative increase in the number of hysterectomies performed for menstrual disorders while the reasons for other diagnostic categories have been relatively stable.

The changing rates for menstrual disorders as a reason for hysterectomy demonstrated in the trend data can only be explained by the interaction of two factors: as a change in morbidity with a constant indication for the operation, or as changing criteria for hysterectomy at constant levels of morbidity. Social acceptance of symptoms may be an element of the second factor. This increase has taken place during a period when many medical therapies are available for the management of menstrual disorders. It could, of course, be argued that the hysterectomy rate would have been higher still if it were not for the availability of medical treatments.

Resource/supply factors

In Bunker's (1970) well-cited paper, he demonstrated that there is proportionally twice as much surgery in the United States as in England and Wales and draws attention to the fact that there are also twice as many American surgeons. McPherson *et al.* (1981) found that 54 per cent of the variance in the differences of hysterectomy rates between regions of England and Wales was explained by the number of general practitioners and gynaecologists. Other studies confirm the direct relationship between surgical resources and rate of operation (Wennberg and Gittelsohn 1973; Vayda and Anderson 1975; Selwood and Wood 1978). These studies provide some agreement with Lewis's adaptation of Parkinson's Law: 'patient admissions for surgery expand to fill beds, operating suites and surgeons' time' (Lewis 1969: 884).

The large international variations in the rates of hysterectomy can in part be explained by the differences in the mode of organization and financing of health services. In fee-for-service systems, such as in North America and Australia, high levels of surgery are performed. The rates are much lower in the lower-resourced centralized systems of health care in Britain and Norway (Coulter and McPherson 1986). While this neat and attractive explanation appears to work at an international level, it does not seem to do so in this case. The East and West comparison in this study produced the paradoxical observation of the association of a higher operation rate with lower gynaecological resources. On balance, it would appear that Lewis's 'Parkinson's Law' is not working for hysterectomies performed in Scotland.

Clinician characteristics

Wennberg (1984) suggested that the type of medical service provided is often found to be as strongly influenced by subjective factors related to the attitudes of individual physicians, i.e. physicians' practice style (which is a result of training), experience, and prevailing medical thought, as by science. Roos (1984b), in a small area variations study in Canada, found that 'hysterectomy-prone physicians' were found to be more likely to diagnose gynaecological problems and more likely to recommend surgical treatment. The effect of prevailing medical thinking on the hysterectomy rate was clearly demonstrated in Canada where a review committee produced a list of acceptable (and unacceptable) indications for hysterectomy which was widely published. In the follow-up evaluation four years later, the hysterectomy rate had dropped by one-third (Dyck *et al.* 1977).

In this study, one of the explanations of the East/West differences is the difference in clinical practice. Although not objectively documented, it is generally accepted that there is little interchange of medical graduates between the two regions of Scotland and there is anecdotal evidence of important differences in clinical practice.

In a clinical decision, the risks and benefits of alternative forms of treatment are weighed up. In practice, however, the scientific evidence required for rational decision-making is often missing (Cochrane 1972). In fact, uncertainty will probably always be an integral feature of clinical medicine (Eddy 1984). McPherson *et al.* (1982) demonstrated that variation for eight common surgical operations between three countries appeared generally to be more characteristic of the procedure than of the country in which it was performed. The procedures for which there was little variation were those where there is a consensus among clinicians concerning their appropriate application, such as appendicectomy. The extent to which variations in rates of hysterectomy related to professional uncertainty is difficult to quantify but it is an important factor.

Patient characteristics

Differences in age composition and age specific disease incidence could be responsible for some of the variation in crude hysterectomy rates in different geographical areas and over time. Age group and diagnostic group analysis for hysterectomies in this study demonstrates real differences and real changes over time. The age standardized hysterectomy rate in the East region of Scotland is 10 per cent higher than the West.

In addition to the above considerations, there is evidence to suggest that there are differences in health care utilization between social classes and higher social class patients ask more questions in the consultation and receive more explanations

(Cartwright and O'Brien 1976). It has also been suggested that some women actively demand hysterectomy; in a *British Medical Journal* editorial it was stated that 'many women today regard hysterectomy as a matter for their decision rather than the doctors' (*BMJ* 1977: 715). Is it, therefore, reasonable to expect the hysterectomy rate to be higher among the higher social classes? Bunker and Brown (1974) demonstrated the higher hysterectomy rate in Californian doctors' wives – an excess of 17 per cent – and which was higher than that for Californian lawyers' wives. Is hysterectomy class led?

In a study based on a Oxford general practice population it was concluded that there was no evidence that hysterectomy is social class related and there is little evidence to suggest that women are either pressurizing surgeons into removing their uteri, or that they are resisting surgery in large numbers (Coulter and McPherson 1986). This study, however, also observed the higher number of other abdominal operations in the patients with hysterectomy. Could this be explained by the fact that these women suffered higher than normal levels of morbidity or are they 'surgery-prone'?

Unfortunately, SMR1 has a high error rate in the social class data, mainly due to omissions. In view of the high error rate of 20 per cent (Table 5.4), analysis of the social class data in SMR1 would have produced misleading results. The occupation data is now no longer routinely collected in SMR1 which is a reflection of the poor validity of this section of SMR1 data.

Artefacts

The regional differences and the trends over time could be due to artefactual causes, for example, systematic omissions of operations due to private surgery, coding changes, and inaccuracies in information sources. The validations of SMR1 and the contribution of private hysterectomy in Scotland have been discussed. It is unlikely that artefacts are a problem in this study.

It is clear from this discussion that the regional differences and changing trends over time of hysterectomy in Scotland are real. This study identifies several research leads for further investigation into this interesting problem which has been described as a 'modern epidemic' (Open University 1985) which has major resource implications for the health service and the health of the patient. Hysterectomy will continue to be an important component of health care in the foreseeable future. Unless we can be sure, on the basis of good research, that for the woman who undergoes hysterectomy the operation is both safe and appropriate, there is a danger that the prediction that Miller (1946) made nearly half a century ago may be realized. He wrote then, 'If what we have observed . . . is confirmed by future studies, then we may be sure that when the curtain rises we shall witness a tragedy, painful and far-reaching in its implication' (p. 810).

Chapter Six

HOW DO YOU COUNT MATERNAL SATISFACTION? A USER-COMMISSIONED SURVEY OF MATERNITY SERVICES

CLAUDIA MARTIN

It is widely believed that research which might influence health policy has to be based on quantitative rather than qualitative data; that numbers rather than words, opinion, or anecdote are deemed more 'convincing' (Wenger 1987). Most of the work described in this book deals with the secondary analysis of large data sets which may, directly or indirectly, affect policy. This chapter is based on a smaller set of data, generated at a local level and intended as a direct response to policy needs. It is rare for research at this level to have a direct impact on health service policy decisions, especially when the research has been commissioned by the users of a service. It is perhaps not surprising that research commissioned by managers may be motivated by factors other than a desire to be better informed about a particular policy issue; for example, to provide reasons for delaying a decision, or to deflect a potential conflict with citizens or, even, within their organization (Hadley 1987).

This chapter describes a research project instigated by a pressure group in the Lothian region of Scotland concerned about future developments in maternity services in the area. The study, a survey of 'consumer' opinions, was carried out by researchers based at Edinburgh University. Some of the findings which might have implications for maternity services in general are presented. The part that the project may have played – or, indeed, *not* played – in influencing local policy decisions is described. Finally, some of the demands, dynamics, and constraints of generating data for policy-relevant research are discussed.

MATERNITY SERVICES IN BRITAIN

In the 1970s, as maternity care was increasingly centralized in large obstetric units, so the amount and degree of intervention in pregnancy and childbirth increased. For example, rates of induction rose from 15 per cent of all labours in 1965 to 41 per cent in 1974 (Cartwright 1979). Caesarean section rates also witnessed a dramatic increase and it is now estimated that one in nine births is by surgical delivery (Boyd and Francome 1983). The number of home births has declined from almost a third of all births in the 1950s (DHSS, Welsh Office 1970) to 4 per cent in the mid-1970s (DHSS 1976a). Fewer than 1 per cent of births now take place in the mother's own home (OPCS 1986c).

These developments, which gathered momentum on the grounds that interventionist hospital confinement was considered safer for mother and baby (DHSS, Welsh Office 1970), appeared to be supported by trends in perinatal mortality. These suggested that, as rates of hospital confinement and obstetric intervention increased, perinatal mortality rates overall declined (Davies 1970). The interpretation that hospital delivery combined with obstetric intervention was therefore 'safer' has been questioned (Tew 1981). However, the factors underlying improvements in perinatal mortality rates are complex and cannot be considered without reference to social and living conditions, the differential risk associated with intended and unintended home delivery, and the selective allocation of 'high risk' maternities to particular hospitals (Campbell *et al.* 1984).

While perinatal and maternal mortality are important considerations in any assessment of maternity provision, such debate has tended to neglect and negate the views, preferences, and experiences of women themselves. There are, of course, some exceptions. Cartwright (1979) carried out a large survey among women who had recently given birth (the survey was principally concerned with women's views of induction) and concluded that many women were unhappy about the care they received; many were not given as much information as they would have liked, and most wished to be more involved in making decisions about their own care. The study also compared the experiences of women having home and hospital confinements and led to the suggestion that ' . . . more needs to be done to improve the qualitative aspects of delivery in hospital' (O'Brien 1978: 460).

MATERNITY SERVICES IN LOTHIAN

The Lothian Region of Scotland extends from the Firth of Forth to a line about 20 miles north of the border between Scotland and England, and meets the Strathclyde Region about half-way between Edinburgh and Glasgow. In addition to Edinburgh, the Region includes a number of small towns, some of which were originally based around the mining industry. Each year there are about 10,500 births in five maternity units in Lothian. The Simpson Maternity Memorial Pavilion (SMMP) in central Edinburgh is by far the largest of the units, dealing with about 4,000 births a year. The other four each deal with between 1,400 and 1,800 births a year. It has been clear for some time that there is an excess of maternity beds in Lothian and, in line with governmental pressure to reduce its budget through efficiency savings, the Lothian Health Board (LHB) has a policy of concentrating in-patient maternity care into fewer units. There are plans for the closure of up to three of the smaller units (all in Edinburgh), to be replaced by a new unit on the hospital site of one of those units threatened with closure. The fifth unit at Bangour General Hospital serves women living in West Lothian.

Widespread concern has been expressed about the proposed concentration of in-patient services. It has been argued by many mothers in the area that large units are more impersonal, less responsive, and place more, and perhaps undue, emphasis on technological forms of care. It has also been argued that fewer units will mean more travelling for Lothian mothers. The three threatened units (the Eastern, the Western, and the Elsie Inglis) have been seen as embodying many of the virtues of smallness, friendliness, and responsiveness. The threatened closure of the Elsie Inglis, in particular, aroused the greatest local disquiet.

Women argued that the 'Elsie's' safety record was no worse than any other maternity unit; that choice was important and that the hospital met the needs of women wanting to give birth in what they perceived to be a low-technology, relaxed, and friendly hospital. However, when the Health Board put forward its case for the closure of 'Elsie's' it argued that this was not a cost-cutting exercise, but was based on a concern about safety. It was argued by the Health Board that the Elsie Inglis was small, isolated, and lacked a special-care baby unit (sick babies are transferred to the SMMP which is about two miles away) and that the safety of mothers and babies could not be guaranteed.

The campaign found expression through the Maternity Services Group of Edinburgh Health Council (the equivalent of Community Health Councils in England and Wales). It was increasingly felt by members of the Health Council that the views of women in Lothian would be ignored in the Health Board's decisions concerning the reorganization of maternity services. At the same time, many of those concerned about the future direction of maternity services have taken the view that the real issue is the *kind* of care received by the mother and her baby – wherever it may be given. Plenty of opinions were on offer about the quality of current services, from both professionals and those outside the circle of providers; but no one could claim to speak authoritatively for the women themselves.

It was at this point, in September 1986, that the Health Council approached us about a possible survey of consumers' views. The research team consisted of myself, Lyn Jones, and Amanda Amos; we are all based at Edinburgh University. I was approached because I have experience of research in the field of maternity services; Amanda Amos, a lecturer in health education within the Department of Community Medicine, is involved in issues of women's health; and Lyn Jones, also a lecturer in community medicine, has an interest in studies of consumer feedback in the NHS.

Preliminary discussions focused around the need for impartiality and independence of any research effort. This meant, for example, that the survey should establish the preferences of Lothian mothers – be it for high *or* low technology births or, indeed, to establish how many women had specific preferences at all. The survey, therefore, had to look at service delivery as it is experienced by women in Lothian, rather than as a vocal and largely middle-class group might like it to be. There was an implicit acknowledgement between ourselves and the Health Council that it was unlikely that the survey would actually prevent closures, but it was hoped that the views expressed by Lothian women would not be ignored in Health Board plans.

Discussions were held with other interest groups – in particular, consultants, nurses, and midwives – and their co-operation and collaboration was sought. The Health Board was then approached and it was agreed that they, with the Health Committee of the Regional Council and the District Councils, would fund the study. It was also agreed that the survey results would be used in forthcoming policy decisions.

METHODS

It was felt that the most efficient way to obtain information from a large sample of mothers, given the financial constraints operating, was by postal questionnaire. Previous research has shown that reliable and valid data about maternity services can be gathered in this way (Martin 1987a).

The questionnaire

The questionnaire covered the following areas:

- antenatal care
- antenatal admission to hospital
- care during labour and delivery
- postnatal care in hospital

Within each of these areas, we asked about the following aspects of care, as appropriate:

- what preferences the mother had
- what choice she was offered
- whether her preferences were taken into account
- accessibility, waiting times, convenience, facilities
- whether she received the information she wanted
- relationships with, and attitudes of, staff
- privacy, noise, food, and so on

We also asked questions relating to overall satisfaction with various aspects of care. Brief personal details were requested, including the occupation of the woman and her partner.

A pilot version of the questionnaire was prepared in the spring of 1987; comments were received on the drafts from the Maternity Services Group and many of the professional staff concerned. The negotiations with each of the groups and individuals involved highlighted their different perspectives and expectations of the study. Thus, the Maternity Services Group were looking to the survey to provide '. . . some kind of evidence to back our belief that although having the right practical support and advice is important, far more important is the overall handling of the woman and her family with regard to emotional needs'. The hospitals' concerns were summed up in a letter from one of the consultants. In the letter he raised an issue of 'acute concern' to him which he felt was missing from the questionnaire, namely '. . . the patient's understanding of the risks involved in becoming pregnant and having a baby'.

In the end, decisions as to what questions to include and how to formulate them were our own. We attempted, however, to incorporate as many of the views and ideas of the interest groups as was feasible. The pilot questionnaire was sent out in July 1987 to 100 mothers who had given birth in April. Responses enabled us to make a number of improvements to the questionnaire.

The sample

Each hospital supplied us with a list of the name and address of every woman who gave birth during a specified seven-week period (1 August to 18 September 1987) – a total of 1,434 women. The questionnaire was mailed in October 1987. The covering letter included, in several languages, an offer of help if the respondent had language difficulties with English. In addition, women whose babies it was known had died or been stillborn were offered a personal interview to describe their experiences, rather than the postal questionnaire. An experienced counsellor was available to conduct any such interview. In the event, this offer was never taken up and most of the women concerned completed the postal questionnaire. Two reminder letters were sent out, at two-weekly intervals, to those who had not responded.

RESULTS

Response Rates

We received 1,107 replies in all; 31 were returned undelivered. This represents an overall response rate of 79 per cent. There were only slight differences between hospitals: the lowest response (77 per cent) was from women delivered at the Elsie Inglis, and the highest (80 per cent) from those delivered at the Western General Hospital. This was a good rate of response and higher than that achieved in a similar survey of three hospitals in London and the Midlands (Martin 1987a). We can only speculate about the reasons for such a high response rate: the questionnaire itself must have been, despite its length, acceptable and easy to complete; women in Lothian may have been motivated by local discussions in the press about the future of maternity services; finally, women may be glad of the opportunity to express their views about an issue which has particular salience for them.

We assessed the representativeness of our sample in terms of age, marital status, parity, ethnicity, and social class against data published by the Registrar General (Scotland) for all births in Lothian (*see* Table 6.1).

Table 6.1 Representativeness of survey sample

Social Characteristic	Survey Respondents (%) (n = 1107)	All Lothian Mothers (%) * (in 1985)
Not married	18	18
First birth (legitimate)	50	43
Age: Less than 20 years old	6	8
More than 35 years old	9	7
Social class IV or V **	27	27

* *Source: Annual Report, Registrar General Scotland 1985*, HMSO (author's analysis)

Note: ** Social class was defined for this assessment in terms of partner's occupation as is the convention in official statistics. There was no information on this for 131 respondents

Compared with all Lothian women who gave birth in 1985 (the most recent year for which data are available), slightly fewer younger and, correspondingly, more older mothers responded to the questionnaire. As the Registrar General only reports the number of previous legitimate births we confined our comparison

153

to married respondents. This showed that the proportion of survey respondents having their first child was higher than for Lothian women in general (50 per cent vs. 43 per cent). Although the survey sample seems to over-represent social classes I and II compared with Scotland as a whole (33 per cent vs. 26 per cent), the proportion of births in Lothian to women in social classes IV and V was 27 per cent which was exactly the same as for our sample. Data on ethnicity could only be assessed indirectly for representativeness. The survey question asked women to state their ethnic origin. However, routine data are available only for Scotland as a whole and refer to country of own birth. Ninety-five per cent of survey respondents indicated their ethnic origin to be 'White/Caucasian' and this compares with an all-Scotland figure of 96 per cent for women born in the UK, Ireland, and Old Commonwealth.

Unfortunately we have no information on the non-respondents, but previous research suggests that postal surveys of recently delivered women may under-represent women in ethnic minorities (particularly Asian women), women in lower social classes, and those whose baby had been ill (Cartwright 1986). In the present study, however, women in social classes IV and V appear to be accurately represented. Thus, although there are small weightings towards older, younger, and first-time mothers, and for women in social classes I and II, these are unlikely to introduce serious bias.

For the purposes of this chapter only selected results are presented. Much of the data analysis concentrated on differences between hospitals and, while these are of interest locally, they are less useful to a wider audience. Therefore, the findings reported here are those which might have a more general applicability to the organization of maternity services. Given the diverse audience for the survey findings, it was felt that data analysis and present-ation should not be unduly complex or technical.

Preferences and choices

This section brings together responses concerning the extent to which women felt they had any choice, particularly over where they had their baby, aspects of their antenatal care, and the course and conduct of their labour and delivery. Women's preferences in

154

each of these areas and how far their preferences were met, were also considered.

Only two-thirds of respondents were offered a choice of where to have their baby. There were, moreover, considerable differences related to social class which largely explained differences between hospitals. Whereas 80 per cent of middle-class mothers reported that they were offered a choice of hospital, only 64 per cent of working-class mothers felt that they had been given a choice in the matter. Social class in this instance was defined in terms of the *woman's* current or most recent occupation. We defined women in non-manual work as middle class and women in manual occupations as working class. In Table 6.1, we used the 'conventional' approach of basing social class on husband's occupation in order to make the appropriate comparison with official statistics.

Six per cent of women had considered a home birth and 4 per cent of the sample asked their GP about this possibility. All met resistance and had a hospital confinement; women having their baby at the Elsie Inglis Hospital were particularly likely to have considered a home birth and then opted for the hospital perceived as 'low technology'. Although 6 per cent might seem a low proportion considering a home birth, it would represent an annual figure for Lothian of over 600 women. In fact, only twelve women had a planned home birth in the region in 1987. We conducted separate interviews with all of these mothers in order to include their views and experiences within the survey.

A great majority (84 per cent) expressed a preference for continuity of care during pregnancy; that is, they wished to be able to see the same doctor or midwife throughout. However, only 13 per cent reported that they saw the same health care professional(s) at every visit, and 33 per cent *never* saw the same person. This seems to be of importance in terms of the women's evaluation of their antenatal care; we found that the greater the degree of continuity of care, the more likely women were to rate their antenatal care, overall, as 'good' or 'very good' (*see* Table 6.2). This finding is, perhaps, not very surprising and is similar to that reported by an evaluation of an antenatal care programme at St. George's Hospital in London which was intended to provide continuity of care for mothers through the 'Know Your Midwife' (KYM) scheme. Flint and Poulengeris (1987) found that women in the KYM scheme were more likely to be more satisfied with their antenatal care and to feel that they had more control in labour than those allocated to the usual system of antenatal care within the hospital.

Table 6.2 Continuity of antenatal care and overall satisfaction

Saw same hospital Dr/midwife	% rating antenatal care as 'good' or 'very good'	(100%=)
Always	87	(128)
Sometimes	80	(533)
Never	75	(321)

Continuity of care in general also appears to have significant implications for the women's satisfaction with communication between them and the health care professionals with whom they came into contact. This is shown in a later section of the chapter.

We asked women whether, before the birth, they had had any preferences about the conduct of their labour and delivery. A set of questions asked about specific aspects of labour and delivery, such as being able to choose the position for delivery, pain relief, and so on, and each question included the options: 'wanted', 'did not want', and 'no preference'. Answers were related to what the women, later in the questionnaire, reported had *actually* happened.

Clearly, some things were seen as more important than others; whereas 78 per cent expressed some prior preference about epidurals only 24 per cent expressed a preference about being able to choose a particular position during labour/delivery. Of course, whether a woman was able to do as she preferred might be affected by unexpected problems which arose during labour or by a change of mind on the part of the woman, and may not necessarily be a reflection of 'obstructive' hospital practices. However, for the most part, women who got what they preferred were more likely to report that labour/delivery had been managed 'as they liked'. This was especially so for women who expressed preferences for low technology options – such as not wanting pain relief, and wanting to be mobile during labour. In general, it does appear that *regardless* of prior preferences, the less intervention there was, the more likely the woman was to feel that labour and delivery had been managed as she wished. Preference for a birth with a minimum of technological intervention is sometimes alleged to be a middle-class predilection. This was not borne out in the survey. For the most part, middle- and working-class women were equally likely to express prior preferences for 'low technology' options (*see* Table 6.3). Social class is again defined in terms of the woman's own current or most recent occupation. Information was not available for 137 women who had either never been in paid employment or who did not state an occupation.

Table 6.3 Low technology preferences by social class *

Preferences	Middle Class (non-manual)		Working Class (manual)	
	%	(N=)	%	(N=)
Considered a home birth	6	(45)	4	(10)
Did not want pain relief	21	(151)	24	(57)
Did not want an epidural	59	(435)	51	(125)
Did not want fetal monitoring	8	(60)	7	(17)
Wanted to be mobile in labour	56	(406)	56	(131)
Wanted to choose birth position	16	(120)	11	(27)
Wanted to use relaxation in labour	88	(649)	78	(182)

Note: * Social class defined in terms of the woman's current or most recent occupation.

Information and communication

Satisfaction with information was strongly related to the relationship between the mother and the professional staff. For example, those mothers who were dissatisfied with the information they received antenatally from their doctor were also much more likely to say that they had been unable to discuss things with their doctor – and similarly for their midwives. This is, of course, what would be expected, but it takes on more significance when related to continuity of care. Women who always saw the same doctor and midwives were much more likely to be satisfied with the information they received than those who saw different staff each time (*see* Table 6.4).

Table 6.4 Continuity of antenatal care and satisfaction with information received from doctors and midwives

Amount of continuity	% satisfied with information	(100%=)
Little or none	60	(106)
Some	72	(381)
All/most of time	82	(457)

Similarly, at the birth of the baby, women were very much more likely to feel they had been looked after with kindness and understanding if they also felt they had had everything explained to them. Table 6.5 shows this quite clearly.

Table 6.5 Amount of explanation received during labour and delivery and how mothers felt they were looked after by staff

Amount of explanation during labour/delivery	% saying they were looked after in 'very kind and understanding way'	(100%=)
Insufficient	36	(53)
Partly sufficient	60	(130)
Sufficient	86	(876)

As an overall indication of women's satisfaction with labour and delivery, we asked them whether these had been managed as they would have liked. More than two-thirds (69 per cent) said they had. However, this figure varied very much according to whether the women felt they had received enough information. Only 23 per cent of those who said they received insufficient information were satisfied with the management of their labour (*see* Table 6.6).

Table 6.6 Information/explanation during labour and satisfaction with management of labour

Amount of information	% satisfied with management	(100%=)
Insufficient	23	(53)
Partly sufficient	33	(129)
Sufficient	79	(860)

Previous studies have shown that there is no social class difference in the desire for information during pregnancy (Cartwright 1979). There is, however, some evidence that, for a variety of reasons, the middle classes tend to get more attention and information from their doctors (Cartwright and O'Brien 1976). The working-class women in this sample were found to be slightly less satisfied than the middle-class women about the communication they had with health care personnel during pregnancy, labour, and delivery. For instance, they were more likely not to be offered a choice of hospital, more likely to report that they did not get enough information, less likely to feel that their preferences had been taken into account during labour and delivery, and more likely to feel that they had not been treated with kindness and understanding. These differences were generally fairly small and not statistically significant, but they were always in the same direction.

A clear and consistent picture emerged from the survey. At all stages of maternity care, the quality of communication between women and the professional staff was a crucial determinant of satisfaction with care. During pregnancy, women who had greater continuity of care were more likely to feel that they had received sufficient information and could discuss things they wanted with the doctor or midwife. Women who were satisfied with the quantity and quality of communication were more likely to be satisfied with their antenatal care generally. During labour and delivery, women who felt they had received sufficient explanation and that they had been treated in a very kind and understanding manner were more likely to be satisfied with the management of their labour.

Perhaps the 'acid test' of the importance of good communication was demonstrated by the answers to a question about where the woman would like to have any subsequent baby. Those who were satisfied with the level of information and communication throughout were much more likely than the dissatisfied mothers to say that they would have a subsequent baby in the same hospital (92 per cent vs 48 per cent).

Differences between hospitals

The responses we received pointed towards some minor differences between hospitals; some provided better continuity of care;

others were more likely to be rated highly in terms of information and communication. Although there were some differences with respect to expressed preferences between women attending different hospitals (the Elsie Inglis, for example, attracting more women who wanted a low technology birth), in terms of women's reports of what happened to them there were, in fact, no real differences between the hospitals in terms of their propensity to intervene medically. None could be characterized as 'high' or 'low' technologically. This suggests, somewhat ironically, that the hospital chosen by women wanting 'natural' births was no less interventionist than the supposed 'high tech' units. Indeed, on some issues such as mobility during labour, the Elsie Inglis was worse than other hospitals; a higher proportion of women at 'Elsie's' (61 per cent) expressed a prior preference to be able to walk around during labour, yet only 37 per cent were able to do so. This compared with figures, for example, of 53 per cent at the Eastern General Hospital and 41 per cent at the SMMP.

One hospital came out, overall, as particularly strong on all aspects of patient/professional communication. This was despite its poor facilities and long antenatal waiting times, all of which were criticized by the women attending the hospital. It was clear, nevertheless, that, from the point of view of users, no single hospital was 'all good' or 'all bad'. Each had its faults and virtues.

Areas of general dissatisfaction

The analysis revealed that there were only a few issues on which a substantial proportion of women agreed that there was room for improvement in all or most hospitals. At the antenatal stage, waiting times in hospital were widely felt (by 30 per cent of respondents) to be unreasonably long, and there was considerable dissatisfaction with having to see different doctors and midwives on each successive visit. For labour, as many as 40 per cent expressed a preference for a room with a homely decor (of the kind sometimes associated with the term 'birthing room'), but only 10 per cent reported actually being able to use such a room. After the birth, over a quarter said that they were not able to get enough rest in hospital – mostly because of general noise levels rather than crying babies. Finally, the most widespread complaint was about the food in hospital, which was judged by almost half to be 'unappetizing', and by almost a third to be insufficient in quantity. Indeed, in one hospital 60 per cent of its patients were clearly very hungry during their stay.

A few mothers had very unfortunate and distressing experiences which contrasted very sharply with the generally satisfactory picture. It is important to remember, however, that when one reports that 'the great majority' of women were satisfied with a particular aspect of care, it may mean that a substantial *number* of women are dissatisfied. Dissatisfaction among 10 per cent of all mothers, after all, means that for 1,000 or more women per year in the Lothian region, there is considerable room for improvement on any particular aspect of care.

In their own words

The way in which most of the questionnaire was framed, coupled with the 'need' for quantitative data, meant answers had to be given in a yes/no or multiple-choice format. We recognized that this might limit the kind of information collected – either by excluding some aspects of the service on which women wished to comment, or by constraining their answers. We therefore left a blank page at the end of the questionnaire and invited women to make any comments that they wished. Over 500 women (46 per cent) took up this opportunity; their comments ranged in length from a couple of sentences to several pages.

The largest single category of comments for each hospital was of those expressing praise for the care and attention the women felt they had received. The women were particularly appreciative of staff who they felt had been working in difficult conditions due to staff shortages or long hours on call.

'Maternity services could have been better in hospital but it was so busy the week my baby was born. If there had been more nurses on duty the care would have been excellent, but this is not the nurses' or the medical staff's fault.'

Several women at each hospital felt that some aspects of the hospital services were being detrimentally affected as a result of shortages of staff and materials, or poor facilities. Many expressed their sympathy for the doctors and nurses who they felt were being overworked and put under considerable strain.

'Care in hospital was satisfactory but due to staff shortages nurses could not give you the care and attention they would have liked. At one point there were three nurses to tend 40 mothers and 41 babies. Eventually mistakes will be made. I feel the nurses did their best under difficult circumstances.'

The proposed hospital closures, perhaps inevitably, provoked a considerable number of comments. The following are typical of the remarks:

'The Elsie Inglis is a very good hospital and the staff are very helpful and nice. It provides a homely atmosphere and you are safe in the knowledge that everyone is looking after you well. Edinburgh will lose one of its best hospitals if they close it. It wouldn't be the same in a wing of a larger hospital.'

'I was very upset to learn that the maternity unit at the Eastern is due to close shortly. If I have another baby I would definitely have liked to go there again. My husband and I both felt that we were very well cared for and everyone was really kind and helpful. Being a small unit meant that you were treated like a human being and not a number . . . '

WHAT HAPPENED TO THE SURVEY RESULTS?

We prepared a variety of reports from the survey. The timing of crucial Health Board meetings prompted us to prepare a preliminary report. This concentrated on inter-hospital comparisons. The second report was a much fuller document and covered broader issues relevant to the planning and organization of services. In addition, each hospital was provided with a dossier containing all the comments which had been made about the hospital, edited to ensure confidentiality. Finally, a report detailing the results of the home births survey (carried out among the twelve women who had a planned home confinement in 1987) has been prepared.

The preliminary report was distributed to the Health Council, the Health Board, and the Regional Council two weeks before the health board meeting which was to approve plans for maternity services. The letter accompanying the report stressed its nature, that its findings were only preliminary, *and* specifically asked that it should be treated as confidential and should not be discussed with the press.

The next day (and in advance of the meeting) the general manager of Lothian Health Board went on national television to announce the closure of the Elsie Inglis Hospital. He then quoted, verbatim, the final sentence from the report as support for this decision:

'There can be no doubt that, whichever hospital they have their babies in, mothers feel that they get very good maternity care from the NHS in Lothian.'

The whole report was subsequently leaked to the press in the course of the following week. Not surprisingly, the parties involved in the research were dismayed; not merely by the breach of confidentiality but by the obvious selective use of the survey research. Selective quotes had been taken from the report and it was quite clear to all concerned that the survey was not going to influence (and probably was never going to influence) the Board's decision regarding hospital closures. The decision to close the Elsie Inglis was, it was suspected, ultimately a financial one. Despite the Board's continuing claim that closure was related to issues of safety, it became known that the Health Board had to save over one million pounds in the next year.

Since the publication of the report, a series of meetings has been instigated between the researchers, the Health Council, the Health Board, and hospital staff to look at the implications of the survey for the staff and the services they provide. These relate particularly to staff shortages and the effect this can have on the quantity and quality of care provided. We suggested in our report that services for the future have to be planned with peaks of activity in mind; that if resources are trimmed, the occasions on which the service is overstretched will become more frequent. This, in turn, may affect the time staff have available for mothers and may diminish the quality of communication with the women. There was ample evidence in the survey that women's overall satisfaction with their care was profoundly influenced by the quality of relationships with health care personnel and the communication that takes place within their interactions – by the continuity of care, the amount of information and explanation, responsiveness to preferences, kindness, and understanding. Although the quality of relationships cannot be built into hospital blueprints or Health Board financial plans, we suggested that they could be influenced, directly and indirectly, by kinds of decisions made at this stage.

INFLUENCING POLICY?

At the outset, it had been clear that each group with an interest in the survey's findings was looking to it to produce data to support their own views. Thus, the finding that, in terms of women's overall satisfaction with care, there were few reported differences between hospitals was open to different interpretations. On the part of the Health Board it was taken as a vindication for closure (that is, as there were no differences between hospitals, it would not matter if one or more were closed), whereas for the Maternity Services Group the finding was taken as an indication of the need to maintain choice.

Carrying out research which one hopes will not only be policy-relevant, but which may influence policy decisions is perhaps an ambitious aim. Obviously, the researchers and the Health Council would have preferred certain of the events which occurred (for example, premature and selective disclosure of the findings) not to have happened. Had our preliminary findings conflicted with the final analyses this could have been very embarrassing. Clearly, it was disappointing to the Health Council that decisions about hospital closure had already been made; this could have seriously influenced already tenuous relationships between the Health Council and the Health Board. Wenger (1987) has suggested that a greater understanding of the differences between groups, arising from research, might, in fact, lead to a channelling of tensions into improved co-operation. This appears to have been one positive outcome of the survey and a dialogue between the two main bodies has evolved.

From the point of view of researchers, the survey required us to operate in different ways and this brought with it advantages, disadvantages, and dilemmas. We were aware that timing was of the essence, that there were a number of crucial and immovable health board deadlines and meetings, and that it was, therefore, vital that the survey results be placed in good time before the relevant committees. With specific deadlines looming, this meant that we had to work in considerable haste. This pressure highlighted the demands of policy-relevant research which, of necessity, limits some of the pleasures of academic discourse. Funding for the study was only £3,500; this figure bears no relation to the *actual* costs. It did not include any payment for our time and, as we all had other commitments, much of the work was carried out in the evenings, nights, and weekends. From the standpoint of the Health Board and the Health Council, it was clearly a 'cost-effective' exercise.

The involvement of 'the public' and health care professionals in the planning of the study promoted co-operation and was welcomed by those involved. In carrying out the data analysis and in preparing our reports, we faced a dilemma: should reports be aimed at the policy-makers, the 'consumers', in the form of the Health Council, or the general public? The form in which findings are disseminated and reported can have important implications for researchers, in terms both of control and credibility with the research respondents (Roberts 1984). Our responsibility towards respondents was an important issue for me. A previous study with which I have been involved concerned the effects of housing conditions on health and was instigated by a tenants' group. A crucial aspect of that study was our commitment to the study and our assurances to tenants that we would remain politically involved with the issue; that we would not merely publish in an obscure journal, but would disseminate findings as widely as possible (Martin 1987b). As with the housing study, the researchers working on the maternity survey were *not* impartial, but the tensions which existed between the Health Council and the Health Board required us, publicly at least, to adopt a neutral position. In order for the findings to be respected by the policy makers, it was felt by all parties that our independence and 'scientific objectivity' were both necessary and important.

Prior to the survey, the Health Board had failed to consult consumers about proposed changes to maternity services in Lothian. While it was galling to realize that certain decisions never were going to be influenced by the survey, one positive outcome has been the development of a better dialogue between the Health Council and the Health Board. The Health Council now has solid data on which to base their views. Because of the leaking of the report to the press by the Health Board, the survey has in fact attained a public profile it may not have achieved on its own merits. The Health Board cannot pretend that the report does not exist and it may, therefore, not be left, like so many pieces of research, to accumulate dust on someone's desk. We would like to think that the Health Board must take account of its contents in the planning of maternity services.

Chapter Seven

WHO'S AFRAID OF THE RANDOMIZED CONTROLLED TRIAL?

Some dilemmas of the scientific method and 'good' research practice

ANN OAKLEY

Randomized controlled trials were originally used in agriculture, and their application to man . . . raises practical difficulties and moral dilemmas. (Dawson 1986:1373)

Human beings are not like grains of wheat. (Faulder 1985:72)

This chapter focuses on the nature and uses of the methodology of the randomized controlled trial (RCT) in the light of recent critiques of science, including the feminist concern with the social structure of science as representing an inherently sexist, racist, classist, and culturally coercive practice and form of knowledge. Using the example of one specific RCT aimed at promoting women's health, the chapter outlines some of the dilemmas thus raised for the pursuit of 'good' research practice. The particular viewpoint from which the chapter is written is that of a feminist sociologist who has been responsible for designing and carrying out a randomized trial in the field of pre-natal health care.[1] While the focus of the chapter is on the use of the methodology of random allocation in health research, it is important to note that it has also been used in other areas of experimental research within the social sciences, for instance in psychology in the evaluation of educational interventions (*see* Rapoport 1985), and in the assessment of professional social work services (Fischer 1973; McCord 1982). Although the study discussed in this chapter and some of the other data drawn on are British, the issues highlighted are of general relevance to all communities where importance is attached to the goal of researching and promoting women's health in the broadest sense.

FROM GUINEA PIGS TO THE CAMEL'S NOSE: ORIGINS AND PROBLEMS OF THE RCT AS A TOOL FOR RESEARCHING WOMEN'S HEALTH

The randomized controlled trial as a research method applicable to human subjects is generally said to have been invented in 1946. In that year, a new drug, streptomycin, was thought to cure tuberculosis in guinea pigs, and initial use on human beings suggested therapeutic effectiveness. Because supplies of the new drug were scarce, the Medical Research Council in Britain decided to administer it in the form of a controlled trial, giving it on the basis of selection according to a table of random numbers to some people with tuberculosis and not to others (Silverman 1980).

Behind this apocryphal story of the origins of the randomized controlled trial lies an intermittent history of previous attempts to carry out unbiased comparisons of the effectiveness of different medical treatments. The RCT is essentially an experimental test ('trial') of a particular treatment/approach (or set of treatments/ approaches) comparing two or more groups of subjects who are allocated to these groups at random, i.e. according to the play of chance. Conclusions about the effectiveness of treatments based on an RCT rest upon two issues – an assessment of *significance* and judgement about *causation*. Tests of statistical significance are used to determine whether any observed difference between trial groups is due to sampling variability or is evidence of a 'real' difference. If a difference is significant in this sense, then, as Schwartz and colleagues put it in their classic text *Clinical Trials*,

> a judgement of causation allows us to attribute it to the difference between (the) two treatments. This is only possible if the two groups are strictly comparable in all respects apart from the treatments given. Providing two such comparable groups is another statistical problem the correct solution of which is obtained by randomization.
>
> (Schwartz *et al.* 1980:7)

It is important to note that the prerequisite for any RCT is *uncertainty* about the effects of a particular treatment. If something is known to work (and to be acceptable and without harmful effects) then there is no reason to put it to the test in the form of a trial. It is, however, this very issue of certainty/uncertainty that

168

constitutes one of the central problems of the contemporary debate about RCTs. People can be certain that something (for example, streptomycin, social workers) *is* effective but have no 'real' basis for their certainty; conversely, unless they are able to admit uncertainty, 'real' knowledge can never be gained.

The RCT has been increasingly promoted over the last twenty years as *the* major evaluative tool within medicine. Over the same period a new critical perspective has emerged towards what counts as 'knowledge' and the methods and techniques appropriate to its accumulation. Sources of this critique include the radical science movement (see for example Rose and Rose 1979), the emergence of 'ethnomethodology' within sociology (for example, Goffman 1968) and the broad consensus located within the women's movement about the 'masculinist' orientation of much scientific activity (Harding 1986). The result of these various critiques has been a heightened awareness of the contribution made by different kinds of research strategies to extending human knowledge in the domain both of the 'natural' and the 'social' sciences.

Over the last twenty years, feminists have increasingly criticized the ways in which the construction of what counts as 'knowledge' omits women's perspectives and experiences and is embedded with masculinist values (see for example, Elshtain 1981; Millman and Kanter 1975; Sherman and Beck 1979). The orbit of feminist concern has included science (Keller 1982; Rose 1983). At the same time as the feminist critique has developed, medical science has expanded its control of life in general and of women's lives in particular. This process has highlighted the need to evaluate all interventions claimed to promote health and has given prominence to the role of the RCT. But, although in recent years feminist researchers have taken to task many methodologies both in the natural and 'unnatural' sciences, there has been virtually no discussion to date of this particular, increasingly advocated approach.

The notion of 'feminist' research, as discussed in this chapter, is taken to mean research that relates to an understanding of women's position as that of an oppressed social group, and which adopts a critical perspective towards intellectual traditions rendering women either invisible and/or subject to a priori categorizations of one kind or another. The research process itself is subject to the same stipulations: that it should not employ methods oppressive either to researchers or to the researched, and should be oriented towards the production of knowledge in such a form and in such a way as can be used by women themselves (Acker *et al.* 1983; Roberts 1981). These strictures are also a formula for 'good' research practice as applied to human subjects in general. However, the practice of feminist research is often located by its advocates on one side of the divide between 'qualitative' and 'quantitative' research methods. Qualitative methods involving in-depth interviewing are seen to be more suited to the exploration of individual experiences – the representation of subjectivity within academic discourse – and to facilitate (in practice if not in theory) a non-hierarchical organization of the research process (Oakley 1981). Conversely, quantitative methods (large-scale surveys, the use of pre-specified scoring methods, for example in personality tests) are cited as instituting the hegemony of the researcher over the researched, and as reducing personal experience to the anonymity of mere numbers. The feminist/masculinist and qualitative/quantitative divisions are paralleled conceptually by a third, that between the physical and the social sciences. As Hedges (1987: 443) has commented: 'Those of us in the social and behavioural sciences know intuitively that there is something "softer" and less cumulative about our research results than those of the physical sciences.'

In terms of this debate about good research practice, the starting point of this chapter is Davies and Esseveld's observation that the problem about the feminist rejection of quantitative methods as necessarily alienating is that it bars discussion both of the ways in which these methods are used, and of those in which they could be used to generate knowledge relevant to the exercise of improving women's situation (Davies and Esseveld 1986: 9). Although feminist research practice requires a critical stance towards existing methodology (the abolition of 'methodolatry' to use Daly's (1973) term), at the same time it has to be recognized that the universe of askable research questions is constrained by the methods allowed. To ban any quantitative (social) science therefore results in a restriction to certain kinds of questions only; this restriction may very well be counter to the same epistemological goal a code of feminist research practice is designed to promote.

According to an Arabic saying deployed by Harris (1974), the problem about letting a camel's nose into your tent is that you are likely then to have to let the whole camel in. The essential question for feminist research posed by the RCT is whether there are benefits of this methodology which can and should be harnessed, without simultaneously dragging into the tent the entire unwieldy superstructure of mixed benefits and hazards (the rest of the camel). Existing published work and the experience drawn on in this chapter suggest that RCTs pose three particular problems for feminist researchers. First and most obviously, there is the principle of *random allocation*, which uses chance – 'the absence of design' (OED) – to determine the treatment received by participants in the research. The extent to which individuals are able to choose the form of their participation in the research is thereby limited. Linked with this is the much debated issue of *informed consent*. What is the meaning of consent, and how much of what kind of information is required by whom? The third problem concerns the epistemology, ownership, and distribution of *certainty*. As already noted, the rationale for undertaking an RCT is uncertainty about the effectiveness/acceptability of a particular procedure. But the professionals may be certain and the lay public not; or the lay public may be convinced about the benefits of a procedure which meets with professional scepticism. It would appear that this issue in particular has provoked a good deal of unclear thinking among those concerned with the promotion of women's health.

Before examining each of these problems in turn, I shall briefly outline the study which highlighted these specific areas of conflict between the practice of *feminist* research on the one hand, and the model of *randomized controlled evaluation*, on the other.

WHO CARES FOR WOMEN? AN RCT OF SOCIAL SUPPORT

The history of the medical care and surveillance of childbearing women is not one of tested and proven effectiveness (Chard and Richards 1977; Wertz and Wertz 1977; Enkin and Chalmers 1982; Oakley 1984; WHO 1986). Studies of how women experience the maternity services have long revealed an iceberg of dissatisfaction, with lack of information, poor communication, long waiting times, and absence of continuity of care coming top of the list (see, for example, Garcia 1982). The complaints women make about their care resonate with an expanding literature on the importance of social support to the promotion of health (Cohen and Syme 1985). It appears (not surprisingly) that friends are as good or better than the famous apple in keeping the doctor away (Berkman 1984). (This may be one instance of modern scientific knowledge catching up with women's experiental understanding of the world (see Chamberlain 1981).)

For these reasons a study of social support in pregnancy was started at the Thomas Coram Research Unit (TCRU) – part of the University of London – in 1985. The broad aim of the project was to establish whether social support provided as a research intervention has the capacity to make things better for women and their babies. Most previous work on this topic is problematic, because of the repetitive methodological problem that, although better health is generally associated with more support, it is impossible to rule out the explanation that healthier, more supported mothers are different in other ways from less supported, less healthy mothers and babies (Oakley 1985, 1988). Although the better done observational studies make multiple adjustments for confounding variables, still one can only adjust for those variables known to confound; there may be others, equally confounding, of which the researcher is ignorant. For this reason, the TCRU study was planned as an *intervention* study, in which the intervention of providing additional social support would be offered to some women and not to others, and various indices of their experiences, including their health and that of their babies, would be compared at the end of the study. Over a fifteen-month period, a total of 509 women agreed to take part in the study. Random allocation was used to determine who received the intervention, and social support was given by four research midwives who visited women at home during pregnancy, offered a listening ear for individual problems, provided various forms of practical and emotional help when required, and were available 24 hours a day to be contacted in case of need. The Department of Health who funded the study were keen for us to have midwives, rather than any other professional or lay group, giving social support because of the study's possible policy implications. The Department expressed the view that, were the study to be successful in demonstrating the clinical effectiveness of social support, the intervention used should be one that related to existing maternity care provisions. In order to increase our chances of detecting an effect of social support, we specified that the women needed to have given birth to a small baby in the past and thus constitute a 'high risk' group. The theory behind this was that women with problematic medical histories would be more likely than those without to benefit from extra support. Additionally, use of this criterion would lead to a largely working-class sample (as two-thirds of low birthweight (LBW) babies but only half of all babies in Britain are born in working-class households), and this concentration of social disadvantage might also result in higher benefit. The 'effectiveness' of this social support intervention in terms of a range of outcomes, including women's satisfaction and infant birthweight, was evaluated after delivery, using obstetric case-note information from the four hospitals where the study was done, and by sending all the women a long and detailed postal questionnaire.

Methods used in this study fit more closely within the medical model of controlled evaluation of therapeutic strategies, rather than with the social science model of qualitative research, in which in-depth interviewing is used to build up interpretative accounts of social processes. However, the study began life as a desire to test the idea that in-depth social science interviewing can in itself have a supportive effect for those interviewed (Oakley 1981; Finch 1984). The midwives giving social support also carried out semi-structured interviews with the women in their intervention group; these interviews were partially tape-recorded in order to enable some qualitative analysis of women's experiences.

CHANCE OR CAUSATION? THE ROLE OF RANDOM NUMBERS

The first of the three problems referred to earlier in combining a feminist research consciousness with the technique of an RCT concerns the process of random allocation itself. We had some interesting and some disturbing difficulties with this. Before discussing these, it is worth considering the history of randomization as a research technique. According to Silverman:

> The central question in the study of living things is how to decide whether an observed event is to be attributed to the

meaningless play of chance, on the one hand, or to causation
... on the other.

(Silverman 1980)

Until the 1920s, scientists were not able to overcome the problem
that very long series of observations were needed in order to
estimate the frequency of occurrence of chance variations. R. A.
Fisher, a statistician working at an Agricultural Research Station in
Harpenden, then devised new techniques for reducing the number of observations needed, by dividing the ground into *randomly*
ordered blocks to be treated in different ways.

As a research technique, randomization is said to offer three
principal advantages. First, each study unit (plot of earth, person,
institution, etc.) has an equal chance of being or not being in the
experimental group. Estimates of chance variability are
consequently much easier to come by. Second, assignment on the
basis of a table of random numbers eradicates the potential for
bias: researchers are unable to influence their results by choosing
to load their experimental group with 'favourable' factors – 'good'
seeds, middle-class women, well-resourced institutions. Third, the
method allows the researchers evenly to distribute both those
factors *known* to be associated with different outcomes and those
which may be, but are *unknown*. An instructive example of the
latter is discussed by Chalmers (1983) in a paper addressing the
competing claims of scientific inquiry and authoritarianism in
perinatal care. In a trial of a cholesterol-lowering drug versus
placebo in the prevention of repeat myocardial infarction in men
(Coronary Drug Project Research Group 1980), no overall benefit
for the active drug was found. However, 20 per cent of those
prescribed the drug had not actually taken it and mortality in this
group was significantly higher, which might lead to the conclusion
that the drug really did work. Researchers then went on to look at
the group given placebo pills: 20 per cent of these had also not
taken their pills and *their* mortality was also significantly higher
than those who had. In fact the group that fared best of the four
(drug prescribed compliers/non-compliers/placebo prescribed
compliers/non-compliers) were men who took the placebo as
prescribed. The *behavioural* factors of 'non-compliance' had an
unanticipated importance greater than that of *physical* risk factors,
and use of random allocation distributed the propensity to disobey

doctors' orders equally between treatment groups, thus permitting valid conclusions to be drawn about the 'real' value of the 'active' drug.

These advantages have led to a characterization of RCTs within medicine and health care research more generally as 'the most scientifically valid method' of evaluating different procedures or types of care (Bracken 1987: 1111). According to proponents of the method, the advantage of random allocation is predominantly *scientific*. It improves the *design* of a study, in part by ensuring that the basic premise – of truly random sampling – underlying the use of statistical tests of significance is correct; in part by clearing the field of unknown 'biases', including those of both researchers and the researched. This removal of the human, subjective element is in line with what Reinharz (1981) and others have described as the 'conventional' or 'patriarchal' research model: research design is laid down in advance, research objectives are concerned with testing hypotheses, units of study are pre-defined, the researcher's attitudes to research subjects is detached, data are manipulated using statistical analyses, replicability of the study findings is stressed, research reports are cast in the form of presenting results only in relation to preset hypotheses, and for approval in an academic community where neither researcher nor researched are allowed identities or personal values. It is, however, worth noting that one of the attributed weaknesses of RCTs – their concern with quantity rather than quality, of life measures – is not a weakness of the method itself, but of its application (see Laing *et al.* 1975 for a counter-example).

Having acquired research funds we then needed to discuss use of the method with those we were asking to use it, namely the four research midwives. In our discussions with them, we emphasized the dual facts that: (a) it was by no means clear that social support was of global benefit to pregnant women (too much social support might be too much of a good thing: at least it was a research question as to which sub-groups of women might benefit); and that (b) we wanted to be able to say something definite about the usefulness of giving social support to pregnant women at the end of the study; use of this method was more likely than any other to enable us to do this. Randomization was done by the midwives telephoning us at TCRU with the names of women who had agreed to take part. The study 'secretary' had sheets of allocations derived from a table of random numbers and she entered each woman in order, then informing the midwife of the result of the allocation.

As the study progressed, we had many discussions about how everyone felt about this procedure. The midwives were sometimes unhappy about both the process and the results of the randomization. They considered it a problem that random allocation was being used to determine which women received additional social support, as this meant that the women themselves could not choose their fates; it also meant that, in agreeing to participate in the study, they were agreeing to a 50 per cent chance of either receiving additional social support or not doing so. Second, the midwives worried because sometimes women they thought were in need of social support were allocated to the control group (standard care) or those they considered had enough of it already were allocated to receive it. One midwife wrote compellingly in a questionnaire we gave them half-way through the study about the conflict between random allocation and the principles of her midwifery training,

'It's very strange in that, if this was practice and not research, you would evaluate each woman and decide if she needed the extra care for various reasons . . . . It's hard if you recruit someone who obviously has major problems and is desperate for extra help, and then she becomes control. I can feel guilty at showing them that extra care is available, and then not offering it to her – even more so if she eventually has a poor outcome to her pregnancy. Conversely, if she becomes intervention and has obvious major problems, I may wilt a little at finding the extra time and stamina to help her!

'It can be a shame if, at first interview, you feel that a woman has no problems, is well-informed and supported, and yet you know you will keep on visiting, when you could spend that time with someone who would benefit more. But it's often not until you visit two or three times that problems become apparent.'

As the study progressed, observations from the midwives about the initial invisibility of women's support needs became more common. The following dialogue occurred during one of our regular meetings:

Midwife 1: 'I think sometimes after the first interview, I wouldn't mind writing down which group I thought they needed to be in. I mean, you see them the first time, and their history's nothing, but when you talk to them, you know how awful it is.'

Midwife 2: 'And it may not be anything to do with their obstetric history.'

Midwife 1: 'Very often it isn't. I went to a lady[2] the other day. On the first visit, everything seemed fine. We were talking away and I got to the section on major worries. She said well, yes, I suppose I have, and it turned out that her older son and her husband, who was not his father, had never got on, which could have had a bearing on the pregnancy in which she'd had a small baby. He'd been in trouble with the police, writing cheques, and so had her son; she brought out all these problems existing in her family since she'd remarried, and she said she can see such a difference in her life now. But I mean that sort of thing doesn't come out at first does it?'

In other words, random numbers have the edge over human intuition because human beings are not always right in the judgements they make. The professional ideology of midwifery, along with that of other health professionals, has been shown to lead to discriminatory stereotyping of women, based on such characteristics as working-class or ethnic-minority status (Graham and Oakley 1981; Macintyre 1976).

The midwives in the TCRU study also tried various ploys to control the randomization process. These included: attempting to spot a pattern in the allocations, so that the order of intervention and control allocations could be predicted, and women entered in accordance with what the midwives thought would suit the women best; and good-humouredly trying to persuade the study secretary to tell them in which order to enter different women (they were quick to realize that the secretary would have the pre-set allocation order in front of her when they telephoned). As well as the factor of women's own needs for social support, the four midwives openly confessed concern about distances they had to travel to carry out the home visits, and about other aspects of their work conditions, such as having to visit possibly dangerous ill-lit housing estates late in the evening. They understandably hoped their intervention group women would live close to home in places which were comfortable and safe to visit.

My own concern as project 'director' on the SSPO study, on the issue of random allocation was, and remained, confused. In the first place, I was committed to the goal of evaluating the effectiveness of social support in a scientific manner acceptable to the scientific community and to policy-makers;[3] this raises its own problems – for instance about the ethics and relevance to women's situation of targeting research at those in power. It is arguable that the usefulness of research in terms of effecting change is greatest when made accessible to the powerless, rather than the powerful. However, the escalating use of unevaluated technology in the maternity care field is a compelling reason for focusing at least some attention directly on those responsible for formulating policy. Because of this goal of reaching policy-makers, I felt it *was* important to carry out the study according to the rules. This, I think was achieved; indeed, our commitment to open discussion of these difficult issues may even have produced greater rigour and consistency in terms of the orthodox model than is normally obtained.

Professional discussions of RCTs are replete with 'anecdotes'[4] concerning people's natural human attempts to control the randomization process. In a trial described by Silverman, for instance, of the effect of artificial light on the occurrence of retrolental fibroplasia (oxygen-induced blindness) in babies:

> Assignment to 'light' or 'no-light' was made on the basis of blue and white marbles in a box. One day, I noted that our head nurse reached into the box for a marble and then replaced it because it wasn't the colour that corresponded to her belief about the best treatment for her babies. I became convinced that we had to shift to sealed envelopes, as used in the British streptomycin trial. When the first sealed envelope was drawn, the resident physician held it up to the light to see the assignment inside! I took the envelopes home and my wife[5] and I wrapped each assignment-sticker in black paper and resealed the envelopes.
>
> (Silverman 1980: 140)

Such revelations draw attention to the discrepancy between the model of 'scientific' research, on the one hand, and its practice, on the other. This discrepancy has been increasingly discussed in recent years, with reports drawing attention to such aspects as the subjective bias inherent in the peer review process (Peters and Ceci 1982), or the tendency for medical researchers to write up and publish research favouring new, as opposed to standard, therapies (Dickersin et al. 1987).

CONSENTING ADULTS?

The issue of randomization is closely bound up with the question of to what extent participants in a research project (either an RCT or any other) consent on the basis of full information to take part in it. The issue of informed consent is the second area of conflict between the principles of feminist research practice and the use of the RCT technique.

In most, if not all, research studies in the social sciences and the market research/opinion survey domain, the people from whom, or on whom, information is gathered are given the opportunity not to take part. This convention accounts for the citation of what, perhaps revealingly, are called 'refusal' and 'non-response' rates: high refusal or non-response rates are considered to call into question the validity (generalizability) of the research findings, whereas low refusal or non-response rates are generally hailed as an achievement for the researchers.

Consent to participate in research is not, however, the rule in medical research, where, according to Faulder (1985), a considerable proportion of the 10 per cent of British patients she estimates to be included currently in RCTs of one kind or another are likely to be in varying states of ignorance about their status as research subjects. The practice of informing people about their inclusion in RCTs appears to have lagged behind their introduction by many years, and to remain uneven between countries. In the USA, written signed consent came into fashion in the 1960s, although more as protection for the doctor than for the patient, given the different organizational base of the US health care system, and its more obvious domination by the practice and threat of litigation.

Until the late 1950s, there was almost no discussion, either in Europe or North America, of informed consent in medical or health research. The term itself seems to have been created in legal circles in 1957, and this legal base has been a continuing important pressure on doctors and medical researchers to consider the issue of what patients should know. In Britain, the current legal position is that, in seeking informed consent, doctors are not obliged fully to disclose all the risks of any procedure, particularly when disclosure is thought by the doctor likely to cause the patient undue anxiety and/or persuade her/him not to accept treatment medically deemed to be beneficial (Brahams 1983). The essential conflict is between what Fader and Beauchamp (1986: 171) term the 'principle of consent' on the one hand, and a 'methodology of deception', on the other.

There is the issue of *what* patients are told; but there is also the issue of *which* patients are told, *when*, and on *whom* data are collected. From this point of view, it is customary to design RCTs in a number of ways. The differences between the designs centre on two issues: (1) the relationship between randomization and consent, and (2) whether or not the trial analysis is done on 'an intention to treat' basis (so that data are collected on all randomly allocated subjects) or only on those who *were* treated. Figure 7.1 shows three variations on the possible combinations of these practices. In Design A, which has been in common use, informed consent is sought only after randomization from the experimental group. However, data are collected on all randomized subjects whether or not their consent to take part in the research was requested and obtained, so that the sub-group of subjects, randomized to the experimental group, who do not give their consent none the less involuntarily contribute data. In Design B, which is the one we used in the TCRU study, consent is sought before randomization. Only those who agree have information collected on them; those who refuse either initially or subsequently are excluded from data-collection and analysis. Since there is no national register of RCTs, it is hard to know the distribution of different designs. However, it would seem that Design C, in which consent is solicited before randomization, but data-collection and analysis proceed on the 'intention to treat' principle, is probably the most frequently used at the moment in UK medical research (Chalmers 1987).

Figure 7.1 Alternative procedures for random allocation and informed consent

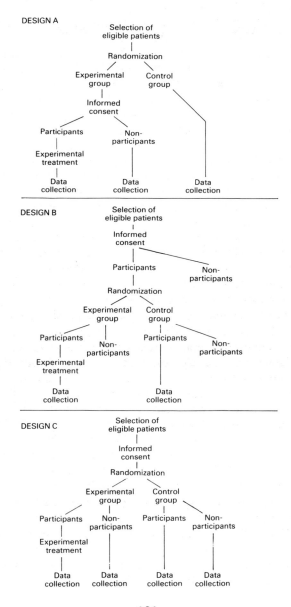

The implications of the different designs for *what* people are told are also quite different (although clearly other factors also influence the extent of disclosure characterizing the consent process). In designs B and C, as opposed to design A for example, what people are asked to consent to is not either to receive a particular intervention or not to receive it. They are asked to agree to putting themselves in a position where they have a fifty-fifty chance of receiving a particular treatment, or not receiving it. In the TCRU study, using Design B, the midwives were asked to follow a text prepared by us, explaining this when talking to the women eligible[6] to enter the study. Women who agreed to take part were randomized and then informed of the result. Twenty-five women out of 534 asked said they would rather not take part in the research. After randomization two women changed their minds – one in the control and one in the intervention group.

Design B is not in common use in RCTs of medical care carried out in Britain. The reasons why we chose to use it can be deduced from the arguments advanced in favour of the other methods, particularly design A. A leading article in the journal *Science* in 1979, 'Informed consent may be hazardous to health' says, for example:

> Before human subjects are enrolled in experimental studies, a variety of preliminary rituals are now required. These include an explanation of the nature of the experimental procedure and a specific elaboration of possible adverse reactions . . . . These rituals are said to increase the subjects' understanding of the procedures . . . .

> A considerable body of psychological evidence indicates that humans are highly suggestible . . . . This alone would lead one to suspect that adverse reactions might result from information given during an informed consent discussion . . . possible consequences of suggested symptoms range from minor annoyance to, in extreme cases, death.

> If protection of the subject is the reason for obtaining informed consent, the possibility of iatrogenic harm to the subject as a direct result of the consent ritual must be considered.
>
> (Loftus and Fries 1979:11)

This is an extreme statement of a position quite commonly stated in the medical literature. The term 'ritual', used in a derogatory sense, immediately tells one how these investigators regard the task of informing people what is being done to them. In another version of this response, the danger that the stress of receiving information may affect health directly results in the conclusion not that *all* patients in a trial should be equally informed, irrespective of group allocation, but rather that *no* patient should be informed at all. Instead, this job is best left to 'ethical'[7] committees, because:

> Only such committees have the experience, skill, information, and emotional detachment to judge the merits of a research protocol; the individual patient has none . . . .

> As a rule, patients will consent to randomization on the basis of skeleton information only, if they know that a committee of professional and other interested people has on their behalf studied and approved the scientific merits and ethical aspects of the trial. Most patients will not need, want, or ask for more.
>
> (Papioannou 1982: 828)

Such a viewpoint invites a number of obvious responses. First of all, reliance on the efficacy or ethical behaviour of ethics committees is dangerously ill-informed. In Britain, no law requires the submission of research proposals to such bodies. There are no statutory or other regulations governing the practices followed in them, which are widely variable, as are the rules controlling membership (British Medical Association 1981).

Second, in the debate about informed consent, the question as to what patients want is rarely constituted as an empirical question, to be settled by appropriate inquiry. Dissatisfaction with the amount and kind of information they are given is the most common complaint patients make about medical care in both the UK and the USA (see King 1986 for a review of this and other areas related to the informed consent debate). A number of studies show that even among people with fatal conditions, over 80 per cent would prefer to know the truth (see, for example, Cassem and Stewart 1975; Aitken-Swan and Easson 1959; McIntosh 1976; for a discussion see Gillon 1987). Studies by Mattson and colleagues (1985) show that among participants in two large trials of drugs to prevent heart disease, increased knowledge was ranked in first or second place as benefits they personally derived from taking part in research. A major finding of these studies was that altruistic motivation ('to help others') was almost as important as the incentive of gaining better care for themselves. Altruism has been an important finding in other fields, including maternity care (Elbourne 1987) and the non-commercial blood donation system that exists in Britain (Titmuss 1970). In the TCRU study, altruistic motives were referred to by a number of the women. Comments included:

'Happy to be of help in getting information to others, and hope to help to improve the system.'

'Very glad to do anything which might help women to cope better with pregnancy.'

'Took part in research to help other people.'

'Quite willing to help with future knowledge for all mothers. Hope it will be helpful.'

'I feel it is very good that things are being researched about childbirth.'

In an interesting account of a 'failed' RCT concerning methods of delivering very low birthweight babies in Australia, Lumley and colleagues (1985) describe how women's reluctance to subject their obstetric care to the play of chance on the basis of informed consent was anticipated by professionals as a problem before the trial started; however, the reason why it proved impossible to carry out in practice turned out instead to be the unwillingness of professionals to subject their behaviour to systematic evaluation. But it is none the less true that research on people's attitudes to information and consent in both health care generally and health research specifically is astonishingly limited. One obstacle is that doctors think patients want to know somewhat less than they do actually want to know (Waitzkin and Streckle 1976). Very little research, for example, has been devoted to the question of how best to give information. One survey of surgical consent forms used in the US found that readability presupposed a university education and four out of five were written at the level of a scientific journal (Grunder 1980). Growing concern about the informed consent issue has now bred the ultimate in RCTs: an RCT of informed consent procedures itself (Simes *et al.* 1986). This compared 'total disclosure' with written consent to an 'individual approach' with verbal consent in patients with cancer who were candidates for RCTs. 'Total disclosure' resulted in more knowledgeable and informed patients who were also less willing to take part in RCTs and were judged to have more anxiety than the less informed group; since anxiety is assumed to be a negative outcome, it is commonly taken to count against the use of 'total disclosure' procedures.

In a chapter advocating the use of RCTs in perinatal research, Bracken introduces two further favoured medical reasons against informing patients when he says that:

> Patients are blinded in clinical trials for two major reasons. First, if blind, they are unlikely to withdraw from an RCT after being randomized into what they believe to be the less effective treatment. Such selective withdrawal would be extremely serious for the success of a trial. Second, blinding the patient avoids placebo effects.
>
> (Bracken 1984: 406)

Not telling people they are part of a research project thus unsurprisingly results in the advantage (for the researcher) that they cannot refuse to co-operate. But what are 'placebo effects' and what are they doing in this argument?

People's belief in the efficacy of what is being done to them has measurable effects on their health (see Brody 1977). Medical professionals hold interestingly divided views on this point. On the one hand, much of the historical efficacy of medical care must have rested on this basis (Ballantine 1975), since, until the twentieth century, relatively few medical procedures could be shown to have any other mechanism of therapeutic effect. The 'placebo' (literally 'I please') response also shores up the notion, close to the heart of many professionals, that the relationship they have with their patients may in itself be healing. These considerations reveal the tension of the physicalist model of health, since it is evident that mind and body interact and that medicine's very claim to effectiveness depends on this, at the same time as disputing it. From a research point of view, however, the placebo effect is nothing more than inconvenient nonsense. A well designed trial must assess it, in order to be assured of credibility.

The giving of information is also said to sound the death knell for the double blind RCT itself. Brownell and Strunkard's paper, 'The double-blind in danger: untoward consequences of informed consent', reports a trial of fenfluramine in 'obese women' in which information given in advance about possible side-effects of medication enabled four out of five patients to guess correctly that they were taking the medication. In turn, this correct estimate was associated with greater weight loss. According to Brownell and Strunkard:

> The implications of these findings are grave: the double-blind methodology . . . can be breached and may be endangered by the demands of institutional review boards for increasingly detailed informed consent.
>
> (Brownell and Strunkard 1982: 1488)

What is highlighted are the consequences for the scientific method of allowing people to know what is happening to them, rather than the therapeutic effect of empowering them with this knowledge.

In the TCRU study, we encountered various difficulties with the method and content of the informed consent procedure we used. Much the most important of these was the extent to which our informing women who were subsequently allocated to the control group what the study was about may have resulted in their feeling deprived (see the midwife's comment, p. 176). One example is this experience described by one of the midwives:

> 'Dawn Benn[8] (Control). She was absolutely desperate to be intervention and she was so upset when I phoned her because of her social circumstances that when she asked me if I knew the address of any mother and toddler groups, NCT groups, anything, because she's just moved into the area, I gave her a couple of phone numbers before I'd even got her allocated. She was heartbroken.'

In other instances, control group women got in touch with the midwives for help even though they knew they had been assigned to the no-support group. We asked the midwives to respond minimally in such situations, conscious that responding fully would be to jeopardize the aims of the study. It is interesting to note that control group women were only able to request this help because the midwives felt it was unethical for them not to give all women in the study a contact address and telephone number. They did so, although this was not part of the study design, and partly in response to our discussions about the informed consent issue.

Evidence of a 'deprivation' response was also gleaned from a few of the women who took part, in the questionnaires they filled in after delivery: for example,

'Pleased to help. I would have welcomed home visits from a midwife.'

'I was very pleased to help, but would have enjoyed the visits . . .'

'Happy . . . (to take part in the research) if it can help anyone in the future. Would have preferred to be in group visited.'

For other control group women, the desire to feel included took such a form that they felt they had been. One of the sections of the questionnaire asked women to tick a list of possibly helpful people, including the research midwife ('if she visited') and thirteen control group women ticked this, though they had not in fact been visited at all. Other appreciative remarks included:

'I wanted to take part and kept a note of how I was feeling at the time of my son's birth.'

'Pleased to have even a small interest taken in my feelings and opinions only inasmuch as feeling I would have some "right to reply" had I been treated very badly.'

'I didn't mind, especially if it helps to understand or prevent premature birth. By filling in this form it helped me to understand any problems I have because I had to write them down.'

One woman in the control group even went so far as to say she felt special as a result of taking part in the research, it was 'like belonging to an elite group'.

Because we gave information to all the women the midwives identified as eligible for the study, the women in the control group *were* part of a research project in which they had *chosen* to participate. In this sense, it is probably true to say that rigorous testing of the hypothesis that social support can improve pregnancy outcome is at odds with the principle of informed consent. A further complication is that the standard scientific model of RCTs presupposes that there is no 'contamination' of the control group by the experimental group; the purpose of the control group is, after all, to act as a 'control' for experiment. (In French, the term for 'control group' is 'le groupe temoin', literally 'witness' group, which carries an interestingly different connotation.) Again, the actual practice, as opposed to theory, of research reveals the chimerical nature of this model. It is assumed, for instance, that people do not talk to one another. In our study, had we not told the control group women about the study, we would have needed to rely on the intervention group women remaining silent about their receipt of social support – at home, with friends and neighbours, in antenatal clinics. But women are not silent. Although this human tendency to communicate may be overcome by randomizing groups (areas, institutions) rather than individuals, the tension between the scientific requirements of research and the humane treatment of individuals remains, and is expressed in the very strategy of designing an experiment so as to restrict people's freedom to discuss with one another the commonality of the process in which they are engaged. A potent example of the scientific disruptiveness of this was described in an RCT of health screening for the elderly in Finland which failed to test the effectiveness of this form of health surveillance, as a local media campaign raised the rate of follow-up examinations in the control group to a figure that was 10 per cent higher than the rate in the experimental group (Antilla and Isokoski 1985).

A second problem we encountered with our informed consent procedure was in deciding how to present the aims of the study to the women we asked to take part in it. The standard procedure for an RCT involves the researcher setting out to test something affectionately known as 'the null hypothesis'. Adoption of the scientific method requires that one begins from the standpoint that there is no difference between the treatment and the lack of treatment, or between the treatments that are being compared. But since we had designed our study to test the hypothesis that social support might affect the baby's weight, as well as to investigate other factors such as the type of delivery mothers had, and how they felt about their experiences, the dilemma was whether we should say so; or if we said 'we want to see if social support can make babies grow better' (for example) were we somehow biasing the study from the start? Might we turn the study into a self-fulfilling prophecy the results of which would never be believed except as such? This formulation of the question is interesting, for it leads to the next question, which is, if the hypothesis is that a *social* process may be therapeutic in a *clinical/physical* sense, what sensible arguments are there for concealing the purpose of the exercise from those taking part in it? The reason why researchers are wary about the placebo response is, after all, because of the possible beneficial impact on someone of feeling they are being cared for: it is the very presence and effect of the social process that is counted as disturbing. But for us the social process was of central concern. It was for this very reason that we decided to enlist the midwives' confidence in the aims of the study from the start: not to have done so would, we felt, not only have been unethical, but also intuitively counter to its aims. For the same reason, we were conscious of the tension with the principle that women allocated to the control group should not feel deprived. Thus, we also stated what we also believed, that we did not *know* whether social support could improve the health of all women and their children in this sense.

THE IMPORTANCE OF BEING (UN)CERTAIN

Third, we come to the last of the issues raised at the beginning of this chapter as especially problematic in this type of research – the question of uncertainty.

Much of the literature on informed consent refers to an uncomfortable prerequisite for the seeking of consent, which is that of researcher or practitioner uncertainty (our not knowing whether social support works). Certainty can be a consequence of very different political and ideological positions. Medical certainty, for example, lies behind one of the most commonly used informed consent/randomization procedures (design A, p. 181). According to Zelen, whose advocacy of this design has been influential, the main advantage of withholding information from the control group is that clinicians do not need to admit to these patients 'that they do not know which treatment is best'. Zelen explains that

> . . . many investigators and patients are reluctant to participate in randomized clinical trials. . . . One of the principal reasons why clinical investigators decline to participate in randomized studies is that they believe that the 'patient-physician relation' is compromised . . .
>
> (Zelen 1979: 1242)

For this reason, use of the RCT is sometimes said to be 'unethical'; the question of ethics enters the medical debate at the point at which the traditional paternalism of the doctor–patient relationship is threatened. From a vantage point outside medicine, however, such professional understandings are precisely the reason why RCTs have an ethical advantage over routine medical practice. They subject to external assessment the medical claim to therapeutic effectiveness (which rests partly on the ambiguous notion of trust). As Freidson has observed, technological/scientific autonomy is *the* premise on which the professionalization of medicine rests; medicine is 'free to develop its special area of knowledge and to determine what are "scientifically acceptable" practices' (Freidson 1970: 83). The aphorism 'doctor knows best' is both a manifestation of this control, and its translation into the politics of the doctor–patient relationship. As Freidson also observes, the *claim* to sole ownership of scientific wisdom says nothing about the *actual* scientific status of the knowledge thus claimed.

However, certainty is not the prerogative of medical professionals. It is also possessed by lay people and by women. The women's health movement has been guilty of a fair amount of misguided certainty over the years, as, for example, in the recently fashionable demand that cervical screening programmes be made more readily available to all women. As Robinson (1987: 51) has noted: 'Neither the ethics, the efficacy, nor the adverse effects of screening have been adequately discussed by women's organizations.' In the childbirth field, many attempts systematically to evaluate different modes of care have been shipwrecked on the rock of women's certainty about the effectiveness of apparently natural and innocuous methods such as childbirth education, vitamin supplements, or raspberry leaf tea. (While such methods may have this effect, there is, as yet, no scientific evidence, and even some to the contrary (see Chalmers 1983).) Perhaps best-publicized of recent examples in Britain has been the response of maternity service user groups to the Medical Research Council's RCT on vitamin supplementation in pregnancy. The trial was designed to test the hypothesis that such supplements, taken around the time of conception, can reduce the chances of a baby having a neural tube malformation. User groups such as the National Childbirth Trust and the Association for Improvements in the Maternity Services contended that the need for a good diet in pregnancy was well established, making the trial unethical (Micklethwaite *et al.* 1982). The point is that, whatever form it takes and whoever professes it, certainty blocks progress towards greater understanding of the role of chance versus causation in the patterning and human experience of events and processes, including those responsible for health or its absence.

Genuine scepticism about something is probably rare. It appears that researchers must merely possess sufficient *un*certainty about something in order to want to find out about it. The issue of certainty was complicated in our study. None of us was prepared to say that we did not know whether social support was a good thing (in the same way as we would have been prepared to say, for example, that we did not know whether it is helpful for women prone to premature labour to be admitted to hospital during pregnancy). But while it may seem almost axiomatic that social support, like love, is something we all want, what is at issue is the range and type of event/process social support is capable of affecting, and the mechanism by which it does so (see Madge and Marmot 1987 for a discussion). Assumptions about the inevitably therapeutic effects of social support may prove unfounded when subject to systematic evaluation. This was the case, for example, in the Cambridge-Somerville Youth Study, an early attempt initiated in 1935 to evaluate the long-term effectiveness of social work help in preventing delinquency and other 'undesirable' outcomes, in which it was found that the intervention of social workers was associated with more problems rather than fewer later on (McCord 1981, 1982).

CONCLUSION

The RCT is a method of *experimental* research, and the term 'experiment' has been linked with what Chalmers (1983) has called the 'Auschwitz' view of scientific inquiry, according to which all experimental research is inherently suspect. The view of experimental research as inherently unethical is central to the feminist critique (Spallone and Steinberg 1987; Birke 1986) but also comes from other quarters (see Silverman 1985). Much of it misses the absolutely crucial point that the condemnation of experimentation under the heading of 'research' allows a great deal of experimentation to pass unnoticed under the heading of standard practice. The frequency with which doctors impose on patients experiments of an uncontrolled nature has been one of the strongest objections to professionalized medicine made by the women's health movement over the last twenty years in Europe and North America (Ruzek 1978). The fact that very large numbers of women have been treated with medical and surgical procedures of unknown or suspect effectiveness and potentially or actually harmful consequences has been taken to signal both women's status as a minority group, and medicine's essentially unscientific standing. For this reason, women have been, and continue to be, important beneficiaries of the advocacy of randomized controlled evaluation within medicine. One significant example concerns the treatment of breast cancer, a disease which affects one in twelve women in the United Kingdom at some point in their lives. Analysis of the results of trials of breast cancer treatments has been responsible for the production of persuasive evidence that 'conservative' treatments are superior to 'radical' treatments both in prolonging life and in assuring a better quality of life. Overviews of RCTs concerned with systematic treatment (chemotherapy or endocrine therapy) of the disease show important differences between the effectiveness of such treatments in older and younger women. They also provide evidence that short courses of treatment are as effective as longer courses – an important consideration, given their sometimes unpleasant side-effects (Consensus Development Conference 1986). It is, however, of interest and important to note that the benefits that accrue to women as a result of their willingness to participate in such studies cannot be held out as a carrot to those who do except by trading on altruism. It is the *future* health of *other* women that stands to benefit by the willingness of *some* to be experimented on *now*.

What our experience with an RCT of social support in pregnancy has shown is the need to subject every precept of the traditional scientific method to scrutiny. Is it necessary? Do its benefits outweigh its hazards? It is as important to ask these questions of a trial of something as apparently harmless as social support as it is of trials of other more obviously ambiguous therapies. The argument against 'methodolatry' is then transformed into the case for an *appropriate* methodology which, like its namesake, appropriate technology, requires that individuals involved in it be treated with sensitivity and respect, and *that there be no division between this ethical requirement and other requirements of the method*. This is not, of course, to say that the procedure of randomized controlled evaluation is the *only* means to reliable knowledge, is *sufficient* in itself, or is *always* the right approach; for the pursuit of truth in human affairs is, as we all know, ultimately an illusion, and reliable knowledge definitely not a good in itself. The point is that what Rowbotham (1985: 51) has called 'the attraction of spring cleaning' should be seen as a means to an end, not an end in itself. The frenetic housewife is unable to enjoy the product of her labours. In Evelyn Keller's words:

> The intellectual danger resides in viewing science as pure social product; science then dissolves into ideology and objectivity loses all intrinsic meaning. In the resulting cultural relativism, any emancipatory function of modern science is negated, and the arbitration of truth recedes into the political domain.
>
> (Keller 1982: 593)

ACKNOWLEDGEMENTS

The original version of this chapter was published in *Women and Health* (Oakley 1990). We are grateful to the journal and its editors for permission to reprint.

NOTES

1. The hierarchy of academia insists on the notion of a project 'director'. However, the Social Support and Pregnancy Outcome study has been a collective venture which would not have been possible without the energy and commitment of: Carol Galen-Bamfield, Sandra Buckle, Rosemary Marsden, Rosie Smith, Lyn Rajan, and Sandra Stone. I should also like to acknowledge the help of Penrose Robertson as the

token man facilitating our use of appropriate technology. I am indebted to members of the National Perinatal Epidemiology Unit in Oxford, and especially to Iain Chalmers and Adrian Grant, for social support, intellectual inspiration, and technical help from (and before) the beginning of the study. Thanks are also due to the Department of Health who funded the study.

2. The midwives referred to the women in the study as their 'ladies'.
3. This raises the question, which is not discussed here, of to what extent the scientific community does indeed practise science.
4. Anecdote means 'things unpublished' but has degenerated to equate with 'an item of gossip' (OED). (And 'gossip' itself is a term which, from describing the important witnessing and authenticating of childbirth by women in the community, is now used in a derogatory sense to refer to 'talk amongst women'.)
5. The role of wives in research, as in other spheres, is revealing.
6. Aside from having had a LBW baby in the past, the women had to be booking into a hospital before 24 weeks of pregnancy and they needed to be able to speak English fluently, as we unfortunately had no money to pay interpreters.
7. An incorrect term. I am grateful to Iain Chalmers for the observation that ethics committees may be ethical – or not.
8. A pseudonym.

Chapter Eight

BEHAVING WELL:

Women's health behaviour in context

HILARY GRAHAM

The election of a Conservative government in 1979 is often presented as marking a radical break in welfare policy. In particular, it has been associated with a well co-ordinated challenge to a consensus about the role of the state in health care, publicly adhered to by the major political parties since 1945. However, in emphasizing the changes that the last decade has brought to health policy, we should not lose sight of continuities. We should be aware of the themes which span the years before and after 1979. One such theme emphasizes the responsibility that individuals have for their own health. Here, it is health behaviour – behaviour affecting health – that is stressed.

The theme was succinctly expressed in the title of the 1976 Consultative Document, *Prevention and Health: Everybody's Business.* Subtitled *A Re-assessment of Public and Personal Health,* it argued that, unlike a century ago, the major health issues of the late twentieth century related not to public health measures but to personal health behaviour. Increasingly, the document suggests, it is the habits of individuals (defined in male terms) which determine the health of the nation. It noted that:

> We as a society are becoming increasingly aware of how much depends on the attitudes and actions of the individual about his health. Prevention today is everybody's business .... Many of the major problems of prevention are less related to man's outside environment than to his own personal behaviour; what may be termed his lifestyle .... To a large extent, it is clear that the weight of responsibility for his own health lies on the shoulders of the individual himself. The

smoking-related diseases, alcoholism and other drug dependencies, obesity and its consequences and the sexually-transmitted diseases are among the preventable problems of our time and in relation to all of these the individual must choose for himself.

(DHSS 1976b: 7, 17, 38)

A decade later, this time under a Conservative rather than Labour government, we find the theme of individual responsibility for health is still strongly emphasized. The 1987 White Paper, *Promoting Better Health*, adopts a less exhortatory style; its language, too, is more gender-neutral. However, like *Prevention and Health*, it points to the way in which the health of the nation is shaped by the behaviour of its people. Like *Prevention and Health*, it sees the major health problems as lifestyle-based: citing cancer, obesity, alcohol misuse, coronary heart disease, and smoking-related illnesses as examples. It concludes that, 'much of this distress and suffering could be avoided if more members of the public took greater responsibility for looking after their own health' (DHSS 1987: 3). It speaks enthusiastically of health education campaigns which 'have encouraged individuals to look positively at their own health and to adopt a more healthy lifestyle', noting that the primary health care team is 'well-placed to persuade individuals of the importance of protecting their health, of the simple steps to do so and of accepting that prevention is indeed better than cure' (DHSS 1987: 3).

The government's message points to the aetiological role of behaviour in health, with the major causes of disease and death in Britain resulting from what *Prevention and Health* calls 'unwise behaviour and over-indulgence' (DHSS 1976b: 31). The message goes further. It suggests that health problems which are behavioural in origin are preventable. The White Paper points to 'the simple steps' that are needed, while *Prevention and Health* states more baldly, 'the individual must choose for himself'.

It is this emphasis on what individuals can do to promote their health – on health behaviour – that is the concern of the chapter. This chapter focuses on how the concept of health behaviour fits within the lives of those whose behaviour may be directed as much to the health of others as to themselves. This focus is developed in the four main sections of the chapter. The first and second sections briefly summarize the evidence on women's mortality, noting how 'unhealthy' behaviour is increasingly seen as the common factor underlying the class distribution of both male and female mortality in Britain. Noting the importance of the concept of health behaviour in the explanation of the nation's health, the third section raises the question of whether the concept of health behaviour can be universally applied to 'everybody'. For example, does the concept have a different meaning for those who are engaged in unpaid and paid 'health work' on behalf of those they care for? Recognizing that it is women who typically find their behaviour directed to the health of others as well as themselves, the fourth section explores the experiences of one group of women: those caring for young children in low income households. Through the accounts that they have given researchers of their lives, it is possible to glimpse something of the everyday meaning of health behaviour for those trying both to 'Look After Yourself' and to look after the family.

INDIVIDUAL BEHAVIOUR: THE KEY TO THE NATION'S HEALTH?

The concept of health behaviour is central to two related aspects of the debate about the nation's health. Health behaviour is invoked as a way of explaining, first, the overall patterns of mortality in Britain and, second, the social distribution of ill-health. In both, the focus is primarily on mortality rather than on the more qualitative dimensions of health: feelings of physical and mental well-being, for example. In the first area, it is the nature and incidence of mortality that have been highlighted; in the second area, it is the social class differences in mortality that have received most attention. While recognizing that mortality provides only a partial (and negative) picture of people's health, both this section and the next follow the furrows ploughed by epidemiological research and briefly examine how the concept of health behaviour has featured in the debates about women's mortality in Britain.

Table 8.1 Principal causes of mortality among women, England and Wales, 1986

Disease	% of total under 75 years	% of total 75 years and over
Coronary heart disease	23	25
Cancer		
breast	9	3
digestive organs/peritoneum	9	6
genito-urinary	6	2
lung	7	2
Cerebrovascular disease (stroke)	10	18
Other (including respiratory disease, diseases of the central nervous system, accidents and poisoning)	37	46

Source: OPCS (1988e) Mortality Statistics: cause 1986

The main causes of death among women in Britain are coronary heart disease, stroke, and cancer (Table 8.1). Personal behaviour is seen as a significant common factor underlying these causes of female mortality. Tables 8.2 and 8.3 below, taken from recent reviews of research, illustrate the extent to which behavioural rather than environmental or genetic factors are seen as 'risk factors' for both heart disease, stroke, and cancer. In the case of coronary heart disease, the leading cause of death in the UK for both men and women, Table 8.2 identifies cigarette smoking as a major 'risk factor'. Cigarette smoking is estimated to be responsible for one quarter of all deaths from coronary heart disease (Royal College of Physicians 1983). Other risk factors are high cholesterol, which is linked to the amount of saturated fat in the diet (Shaper *et al.* 1985), and high blood pressure, where 'genetic factors, obesity, heavy drinking, and high dietary salt intake probably all play a part' (Smith and Jacobson 1988: 34).

The second leading cause of death in Britain among men and women is cancer. Reviewing the evidence on cancer mortality, Smith and Jacobson concluded in their review of *The Nation's Health* that, 'although we do not yet know enough about the causes of cancer, the two most important – cigarette smoking and diet – stand out clearly against the background of risk factors' (Smith and Jacobson 1988: 44). As Table 8.3 indicates, research suggests that one third (35 per cent) of cancer deaths are attributable to diet, with a further third (30 per cent) attributable to smoking (Doll and Peto 1981). Looking at specific forms of cancer, behavioural factors are again strongly emphasized. 90 per cent of all lung cancer mortality has been linked to cigarette smoking (Royal College of Physicians 1983). In bowel cancer, diet has been singled out, while sexual behaviour is seen as important in the aetiology of cervical cancer. However, in relation to breast cancer, health behaviour is less obviously implicated. Here, an early age of menarche and a first pregnancy after the age of 35 years both appear as 'risk factors'.

Table 8.2 Known risk factors for coronary heart disease and stroke (men and women)

Risk Factor	Relationship to CHD
'classical' risk factors	
cigarette smoking	causal
high blood cholesterol	causal
high blood pressure	causal
other risk factors	
obesity	possibly causal
diabetes	probably causal
physical inactivity	probably causal
social class	independent association
psychosocial factors	strong independent association
heavy alcohol consumption	strong independent association
soft tap water	association
family history	strong association

Source: adapted from A. Smith and B. Jacobson (1988) *The Nation's Health*, Table 2, p. 30

While female mortality from coronary heart disease and cancer has been, and remains, lower than male mortality from these diseases, recent decades have seen a narrowing of the traditional sex differentials in death rates. Since the mid 1970s, there has been a decline in mortality from coronary heart disease among both men and women. However, the reduction between 1978 and 1986 among men aged 55–74 was more than twice that observed for women (N. Wells 1987). Lung cancer rates among men fell over the two decades from 1963: during the same period, lung cancer rates among women doubled (Smith and Jacobson 1988). Reflecting this pattern, the sex differential in lung cancer mortality has been steadily closing through the 1970s and 1980s. Turning to breast cancer, rates of female mortality have changed little over the last decade. The trend, if anything, has been towards a slight increase in mortality (Wells 1989).

Table 8.3 Proportion of cancer deaths attributable to different factors (men and women)

Factor or class of factors	% of all cancer deaths: best estimate
diet	35
tobacco	30
reproductive and sexual behaviour	7
alcohol	3
	75
infection	10 ?
occupation	4
geophysical factors	3
pollution	2
medicines and medical procedures	1
industrial products	<1
food additives	<1
unknown	?
	22 ?

Source: adapted from R. Doll and R. Peto (1981) 'The causes of cancer', *Jnl. of the National Cancer Institute,* 66, pp. 1191–308

Again, it is 'lifestyle factors' that are seen to play a significant role in these trends. For example, one recent review of women's mortality identified:

> coronary heart disease, stroke, breast and lung cancer as major causes of premature death among women. These diseases and many others are causally associated with lifestyle factors . . . . A consistent aspect of the four principal causes of premature female death is the established or suspected role played by a number of factors connected with lifestyle. Cigarette smoking, excess alcohol consumption, inappropriate diet and lack of exercise – the key influences – are of course also linked to many other diseases.
>
> (N. Wells 1987: 67, 65)

As this comment indicates, personal behaviour is seen to explain, at least in part, the patterns of female mortality in the UK. The aetiological significance of personal behaviour, however, extends beyond debates about sex differences in mortality. Personal behaviour is also seen to hold the key to understanding other dimensions of the social distribution of health, and to understanding the marked social class differences in mortality in particular.

INDIVIDUAL BEHAVIOUR: THE KEY TO THE SOCIAL CLASS DISTRIBUTION OF HEALTH?

To a greater extent than in some other European countries, health in Britain follows the contours of social disadvantage. Rates of morbidity and mortality are higher among people in working-class households than among those who live in middle-class households (OPCS 1986a; Marmot and McDowall 1986) and they are higher in the economically deprived areas of Britain than in the more affluent districts (Townsend 1987; Hyde *et al* 1989). Because of the way in which women's class position is measured, it is more difficult to interpret the links between social class and mortality for women than it is for men. In an attempt to overcome these problems, Moser *et al* re-examined mortality data using information on women's marital status, own occupation, economic activity, and household wealth (housing tenure and access to a car) in addition to partner's occupation (if married). Their analysis suggested that high mortality among women was associated with working in a manual occupation, being a single woman in a manual occupation, living in a rented house, and having no access to a car (Moser *et al* 1988a). Where these indicators of disadvantage were combined, they found that mortality rates were two to three times higher than for women with none of these disadvantages. Thus, for single women in households with a car and in non-manual jobs, the SMR was 69: for single women in manual jobs and living in households without access to a car it rose to 178. This approach is discussed in more detail in the chapter by Helena Pugh and Kath Moser.

Black and ethnic minority women are particularly likely to experience those forms of multiple and reinforcing disadvantage associated with high mortality rates (Brown 1984). However, there are few sources of data which shed light on their health experiences. Taking country of birth as a proxy measure, OPCS data suggest that women born in the New Commonwealth (Indian sub-continent, Caribbean Commonwealth, and the African Commonwealth) have higher rates of mortality, including markedly higher rates of maternal mortality, than other women (Marmot *et al.* 1984; Grimsley and Bhat 1988). Their children, too, are more vulnerable to premature death (Terry *et al.* 1980; OPCS 1985a).

It is not only health that varies with social position: health behaviour does too. The 'risk factors' associated with both heart disease and cancer tend to be more common among those living in working-class households and among those living in the north of England. The patterns of women's smoking are summarized in Table 8.4, which suggests that three times as many women in unskilled manual households smoke cigarettes as those in households classified as professional. The proportion of smokers is higher, too, in the north of England, in Wales, Scotland, and Northern Ireland than it is in the south of England (OPCS 1989a). While smoking is strongly linked to social disadvantage, it is not associated with racial disadvantage. Black women (Afro-Caribbean and Asian) are more likely to live in the social classes and regions of Britain where disadvantage is clustered (Brown 1984). Yet, while they are particularly vulnerable to the disadvantages that are linked to smoking among white women, only a small proportion of black women are smokers (Graham 1988). Smoking, and heavy smoking in particular, has a strong racial identity as a white health behaviour.

Table 8.4 Women's smoking status by household socio-economic group
(1985)

Household socio-economic group	% current regular smokers
professional	14
employers/managers	28
other non-manual	26
skilled manual	35
semi-skilled manual	37
unskilled manual	45

Source: John Golding in B.D. Cox *et al.* (1987) *The Health and Lifestyle Survey,* Table 10.3

The evidence on diet suggests that individuals in households in the higher income brackets have a healthier diet than those living in households on low incomes. Data on two indicators of a 'healthy diet' – the consumption of brown bread and fruit – are summarized in Tables 8.5 and 8.6. While richer households consume more fresh fruit and vegetables and brown bread, poorer households consume significantly more white bread, sugar, potatoes, and fats (DE 1988). Again, we know relatively little about the diets of black women within these socio-economic groups, with the limited sources of information deriving from small, local studies (Homans 1983; Wheeler and Tan 1983; McKeigue *et al.* 1985).

Table 8.5 Percentage of women aged 18–49 who usually consume 'brown' bread by household socio-economic group (1985)

Household socio-economic group	% usually consuming brown bread
professional	72
employers/managers	56
other non-manual	54
skilled manual	40
semi-skilled manual	34
unskilled manual	30

Source: Margaret Whichelow in B.D. Cox *et al.* (1987) *The Health and Lifestyle Survey*, Table 8.8

Table 8.6 Percentage of women aged 18–39 who consume fruit every day in summer by household socio-economic group (1985)

Household socio-economic group	fruit consumed every day
professional	74
employers/managers	73
other non-manual	64
skilled manual	59
semi-skilled manual	54
unskilled manual	42

Source: Margaret Whichelow in B.D. Cox *et al* (1987) *The Health and Lifestyle Survey*, Table 8.13

It is the complex associations between social class, individual behaviour, and mortality which are at the heart of the so-called 'health inequalities debate'. While suggesting a broadly focused discussion of the way social divisions – of gender, race, social class, and region – are reflected in the health experience of individuals, 'health inequalities' have been more narrowly defined in terms of social class differences. The debate – most recently reviewed in *The Health Divide* (Townsend *et al.* 1988) – is thus concerned with how the social class differences in mortality might be explained. While a range of explanations has been proposed, the debate over the last decade has focused on two perspectives, somewhat crudely identified as the cultural/behavioural and material/structural perspectives.

A cultural/behavioural perspective suggests that the class-related patterns of health reflect cultural differences in how individuals live. Here, individual lifestyles are seen as moulded by the values and accepted patterns of behaviour within the wider communities of which the individual is a member. This explanatory model points to the opportunities for change: through instilling a greater knowledge of and responsibility about health. It is this cultural/behavioural perspective which informs the two government documents considered at the beginning of the chapter: *Prevention and Health*, with its message that 'the weight of responsibility for his own health lies on the shoulders of the individual himself' (DHSS 1976b) and *Promoting Better Health*, with its concern that people take 'greater responsibility for looking after their own health'. It is a perspective more succinctly summed up by Edwina Currie in her observation that northerners are 'dying of ignorance and chips', while '*Independent* and *Guardian* readers have bean sprouts coming out of their ears'.

While the material/structural model recognizes social class differences in health behaviour, it sets health behaviour alongside and in the context of the everyday circumstances in which people live and work. Thus, alongside behavioural factors, attention is drawn to the adverse effects of material deprivation on health: to the physical environment of the home and the workplace, and to the restrictions on diet and heating that poverty brings. Attention is also drawn to other forms of social disadvantage, including those linked to gender and 'race' (Graham 1984; Bhat *et al.* 1988). It is these factors that are seen to shape and constrain what individuals can do to promote their health, setting limits on the choices they can make about their lifestyle.

Within this structural perspective, the separation of 'structure' and 'behaviour', of living conditions and lifestyles, tends to dissolve. It is living conditions which are seen to provide the context in which lifestyles are sustained (Blaxter 1983; Blane 1985). In suggesting that the distinction between social and behavioural factors is an artificial one, questions have been raised about the aetiological role ascribed to 'health behaviour'. Some researchers have questioned whether a strong statistical relationship between the two components of the concept – between health and behaviour – can be taken as proof of a strong causal one. The argument is usually expressed in cautious terms. The suggestion made is that the association may not be as strong as the epidemiological evidence indicates. The argument turns on the relative difficulties of measuring social conditions and individual behaviour. It is difficult to unravel and to measure the complex and changing elements of an individual's environment and, as a result, as Wilkinson observes, 'class often serves as an undefined proxy for the effects of unknown socio-economic differences, (Wilkinson 1986: 18). By comparison, the identification and measurement of an individual's behaviour within this environment is relatively straightforward. Further, because behaviours like smoking are class-related, those who are exposed to the health risks of smoking are also likely to be exposed to other health hazards that vary in systematic ways with social class (Blane 1985).

As a result of these problems of measurement, health behaviours like cigarette smoking may be 'standing in', at least in part, for social class. While the evidence suggests that health behaviour *is* independently related to health (Fogelman 1980; Marmot 1986), some of the health-effects ascribed to behaviour may derive from cumulative material disadvantages experienced over a lifetime.

In the sections that follow, the complex links between living conditions and lifestyles are explored further. Here, it is the material/structural perspective which is seen to offer particular insight into women's everyday experiences of pursuing health through their behaviour. While beliefs, knowledge, and motivations clearly shape routines, women's accounts of their lives point to ways in which the social and material conditions of caring act as a brake on how far health principles can be translated into health practices.

BEHAVING WELL FOR OTHERS: CARING AND THE CONCEPT OF HEALTH BEHAVIOUR

The concept of health behaviour carries a generalized health warning about what we can do to damage (and promote) our own health. The focus is the individual: an activity earns the label 'health behaviour' if it is associated with a reduced or increased incidence of a particular disease for the individual who engages in it (as, for example, indicated in Tables 8.2 and 8.3). While the individual is the unit of analysis in most studies of health and behaviour, there are some important exceptions. One major example is passive smoking: the involuntary inhalation of other people's smoke. Here, it is recognized that the analysis must be extended to include those affected by an individual's health behaviour. In relation to passive smoking, the most well-researched dyad is the mother and her (unborn) child (Fogelman and Manor 1988). The perspective in such research is broader, encompassing two individuals rather than one. However, behaviour is still assessed in one-dimensional terms, as either 'healthy' (not smoking, going to the ante-natal clinic) or 'unhealthy' (smoking, being a non-attender).

While the individual is the focus in much epidemiological research, the evidence from sociological studies suggests that many people assess their health behaviour in a less individualistic way. Research indicates that it is women, in particular, who tend to define their behaviour in terms of the health of others as well as themselves (Cornwell 1984; Pill and Stott 1985). Women's propensity to see health behaviour as a multi-dimensional concept is linked, in turn, to the fact that women's lives tend to be structured by their responsibilities for the health of others. It is therefore by exploring the lives of women that we can begin to grasp some of the complexities of health behaviour.

Estimates suggest that more than 1.4 million people are engaged in the informal care of a sick, disabled, or older person, devoting more than 20 hours a week to health-related tasks (OPCS 1988d). In addition, there are 8 million households with children under 15. Here, the evidence suggests that, in the majority of households, one parent takes on the role of health-provider, adapting their everyday routines and habits to meet the health needs of their children and partners as well as themselves. One study of childcare suggested that the 'principal carer' of able-bodied children under two years of age spent eight hours a day in health behaviours directed towards their children: getting children up and dressed, toileting, feeding, bathing, etc. (Piachaud 1985).

Like other types of work, 'health work' is tied into the social divisions which characterize British society. As unpaid work, working for health has a strong gender identity as women's work. Among those providing at least 20 hours of personal care for older people, disabled people, and those suffering from long-term illness, research suggests that over 60 per cent are women (OPCS 1988d). Among those caring for children about three out of every four women in households with pre-school children are full-time carers (OPCS 1989a). Among parents caring for children alone, women outnumber men nine to one. It is not only tasks directly connected with the health of dependent people that tend to be done by women. Domestic work, much of it health related, also displays this strong sexual division of labour. As Table 8.7 suggests, women, even when they work full-time, do most of the day-to-day health work on behalf of both themselves and their partner.

Table 8.7 Domestic division of labour by sex and working status of women (1987)

Household tasks	Man works/ woman works full-time	Man works/ woman works part-time	Man works/ woman not employed
makes evening meal			
mainly man	7	4	1
mainly woman	63	83	89
shared equally	28	13	10
does household cleaning			
mainly man	4	1	1
mainly woman	60	84	86
shared equally	33	14	11
does washing and ironing			
mainly man	1	–	2
mainly woman	81	94	93
shared equally	18	5	5

Source: R. Jowell, S. Witherspoon, and L. Brook, (1988) *British Social Attitudes: the 5th Report*, Gower, Aldershot, Hants

The experience of taking responsibility for the health care of others – and members of the family in particular – is a ubiquitous part of women's lives in Britain. Most women live with men (74 per cent of women aged 18 to 49 years were married or cohabiting in 1985) and most women become mothers (EOC 1988). An indirect measure of the impact of the 'health work' of marriage and motherhood on women is provided by the statistics on paid employment. Married women – even when they have no young children – are less likely to be in full-time employment and more likely to be in part-time employment than those living on their own. Mothers with pre-school children are unlikely to have paid jobs, while those with older children are likely to work only part-time (Joshi 1986).

Turning from unpaid to paid health-work, we find that not only is it 'gendered' work, it is also work which is racially structured and class-divided. Overall, 11 per cent of white women in paid employment work in the health services (state and private); among black and ethnic minority women the proportion is 17 per cent (Ohri and Faruqi 1988). Looking specifically at the National Health Service, about 75 per cent of its workforce are women; among nurses, the proportion rises to over 90 per cent (Doyal 1985). Within this female workforce, ethnic minority women are disproportionately represented in the lower status and lower paid positions: in geriatric and psychiatric care, in the SEN grades and in ancillary work. A study of one London hospital found that 80 per cent of those employed in ancillary, domestic, and catering grades were born overseas (Doyal *et al.* 1981). A similarly structured labour force services the American health care system. In the USA, most health care workers are women (72 per cent) and non-white (69 per cent), while most administrators are male and white (Coleman and Dickenson 1984).

It is thus those in the more disadvantaged positions in our social structure who are most likely to combine health behaviour with health work. It is women rather than men, black rather than white, working class rather than middle class who are most likely to be combining health behaviour (for themselves) with health work (for others). Where their daily lives have this multi-dimensional quality, the assessment of behaviours as health promoting or health damaging may be a more complex exercise than the epidemiological evidence suggests. Set in the context of everyday life, the question of what promotes and what damages health may become more ambiguous and more contradictory. It is this question that is explored in the section below, where the focus is on mothers caring in poverty.

BEHAVING WELL: WOMEN'S EXPERIENCES OF HEALTH BEHAVIOUR IN POVERTY

The concept of health behaviour – as behaviour with an effect on our health – is not only one recognized by social scientists and policy makers. It is also a concept which has widespread public support. Table 8.8 suggests that women are more likely to see individual behaviour, rather than the external environment, as the primary determinant of their own health. Looking at specific types of behaviour, the Health and Lifestyle Survey found that the majority of women identify smoking as a cause of lung cancer (84 per cent) and bronchitis (53 per cent); a quarter (25 per cent) identified it as a cause of heart attacks (Cox *et al* 1987). These patterns, which are consistent with other studies of health beliefs (Marsh and Matheson 1983), suggest that the lifestyle message has been absorbed and accepted by a significant proportion of women. The barriers to 'behaving well', it appears, are not simply ones relating to knowledge about the health consequences of behaviour.

Table 8.8 The relative importance given to voluntary behaviours, environmental causes outside one's control and psycho-social factors affecting one's own health : women (1985)

Household socio-economic group	Importance given to *		
	behaviour in one's control %	environmental factors outside one's control %	psycho-social factors %
professional/ employer/manager	43	22	38
other non-manual	41	17	30
skilled manual	35	16	30
semi-and unskilled manual	35	15	29
all women	38	18	32

Source: Mildred Blaxter in B.D. Cox *et al.* (1987) *The Health and Lifestyle Survey*, Table 14.6
Note: * a respondent may appear in more than one category, or none of these

In seeking to understand more about women's health behaviour, this section explores the everyday experiences of women caring for children in low income households. It focuses, first, on the experience of caring in poverty, turning, second, to particular patterns of health behaviour associated with low income households. The discussion draws on a study of 57 mothers caring for pre-school children which I conducted in 1984 (Graham 1986). The households were either living on supplementary benefit, or had incomes which were at or below the level of supplementary benefit. Reflecting the area in which the study was based, most of the mothers (90 per cent) were white.

While the experiences of one small group of mothers cannot be generalized to 'all women', embedded within these experiences are features which, perhaps in a less sharp form, shape the lives of many women. The experience of living (and caring) in poverty is one that is more common among women than men in Britain. Women are over-represented in those households particularly vulnerable to poverty: pensioner households and lone parent households, for example (Glendinning and Millar 1987). Research also suggests that women are more vulnerable than men to poverty resulting from the inequitable distribution of resources within households (Homer *et al.* 1984; Graham 1987a; McKee 1987; Pahl 1988). Its invisibility makes the extent of 'hidden' poverty hard to estimate, but its existence reminds us that we need to explore how the poverty of, and the poverty within, households structures health behaviour if we are to understand the problems women may face in 'behaving well'.

Caring in poverty

Estimates of the number of people living in poverty can be derived from the government's statistics of low income families (DHSS 1988b). If we take the level of supplementary benefit as our poverty line, these statistics suggest that, in 1985, there were 4 million people in households with children living on incomes on or below the poverty line/supplementary benefit level. Another 2.4 million were living on incomes up to 40 per cent above the level of supplementary benefit (DHSS 1988b). These figures suggest that one in five mothers living with a partner are caring for children in low income households (up to 40 per cent above the level of supplementary benefit/income support). Among lone mothers, the proportion rises to three in four (74 per cent).

While the concepts of absolute and relative poverty are generally defined in terms of household income rather than individual living standards, both concepts shed light on the health behaviour of mothers within these low income households. Health is built into the definition of absolute poverty (Rowntree 1902). As B. S. Rowntree put it, living below the poverty line means living on an income 'below the minimum sums on which families of different sizes could be maintained in a state of physical efficiency' (Rowntree 1903, quoted in Veit-Wilson 1986). In households at the poverty line, life is governed by the regulation, 'nothing must be bought but what is absolutely necessary for the maintenance of physical health' (Rowntree 1941: 103). An absolute conception of poverty thus alerts us to the fact that health – for some or all of the family – may need to be bartered in the struggle to make ends meet.

A relative definition of poverty highlights not only the physical effects of living close to or below the subsistence level. It also alerts us to the psychological and social consequences of having to live, not through choice, outside the day-to-day cultural and political life of the community. As Townsend notes, 'individuals, families and groups can be said to be in poverty when . . . their resources are so seriously below those commanded by the average individual or family that they are, in effect, excluded from ordinary living patterns, customs and activities' (Townsend 1979: 31). As Townsend's definition suggests, a relative concept of poverty points to the social isolation of the poor. It alerts us to their enforced privacy and their restricted access to a world which, if available, could compensate for the material privations of the home.

Taking an absolute view of poverty, the figures on low income draw our attention to the numbers of parents and children for whom health may be under direct threat. Taking a relative view of poverty, the figures point to a significant minority of households unable to participate in the lifestyles and social activities which the majority take for granted. This definition highlights the important issues of social exclusion and economic disenfranchisement from the normal experiences of parenthood and childhood, issues we return to below.

As the person who typically assumes responsibility for day-to-day budgeting and for day-to-day health care, it is often the mother who feels most acutely the conflicts between housekeeping and health keeping on a low income. These conflicts are reflected in the budgeting patterns found among low income households. Low income households typically prioritize collective items essential for the health and survival of the family: housing, fuel, food. Items of expenditure deemed non-essential and individual are restricted. This pattern of priorities is reflected in Table 8.9, which compares the absolute and relative amounts spent on different items of expenditure by households with children (excluding housing costs). It indicates that the family on supplementary benefit devotes more of its weekly income to food (41 per cent) and fuel (15 per cent) than the average for all households with two adults and two children. Overall, over half (56 per cent) of their weekly income goes on these two basic necessities: the average proportion is under a third (31 per cent). The one major exception to the budgeting strategy of low income families is tobacco (Graham 1988). As Table 8.9 suggests, relative spending on tobacco is higher in the family on supplementary benefit. This is an issue explored in more depth below.

Table 8.9 Weekly expenditure for two-adult, two-child households: average of all households and a household on supplementary benefit (SB), 1986

| | Average household | | SB | |
	£	%	£	%
fuel	12	7	11	15
food	45	24	31	41
clothes/footwear	17	9	4	5
durable household goods	20	11	3	4
transport	30	16	5	7
services	25	13	5	7
alcohol	9	5	2	3
tobacco	5	3	5	7
Total	186		75	

Source: Adapted from *Budgeting on Benefit: the Consumption of Families on Social Security* by Jonathon Bradshaw and Jane Morgan (1987) London, Family Policy Studies Centre

Within – or in conflict with – this system of priorities, financial commitments to outside agencies are met first. Rent, rates, fuel bills, and debt and hire purchase repayments thus tend to have first call on the household income. Despite the priority given to 'the bills', many households have difficulty meeting external commitments. One in five low income households with children have arrears for either gas or electricity or both (Hutton 1986). Fuel and other household debts are more common among households with children (Parker 1988). In one recent study of 64 households with children living on benefit, 95 per cent were found to be in 'substantial debt'. 30 per cent of the sample had debts of over £500 (Holmes 1988).

The system of financial management, where payments to outside agencies are prioritized, has particular implications for those with responsibility for meeting health needs. Paying fixed costs first helps to secure some important health resources like housing and heating. But it means that spending on other resources directly related to health and child development – including food, clothes and shoes, public transport to social and health facilities, playgroup expenses, and toys – is severely restricted. It is the food budget that is most clearly affected: it is the largest single item of weekly expenditure (see Table 8.8) and, unlike most other items of collective health expenditure, it is not purchased through one lump-sum payment to an outside agency. It is also the largest item over which the mother is likely to exercise direct control. It is here, in the diet which she provides her family, that the struggle against poverty is most likely to be felt. Mothers bringing up their children on supplementary benefit explained the implications for family feeding in these terms:

> Food's the only place I find I can tighten up. The rest of it, they take it before you get your hands on it really. So it's the food . . . . The only thing I can cut down is food . . . . You've got to balance nutrition with a large amount of food that will keep them not hungry. I'd like to give them fresh fruit, whereas the good food has to be limited.

> I usually just have to buy the same things each week. You know what I mean, it's a routine. It's all you can afford. I know you should think about what's good for you. I do *think* about it. But there again, you can't *do* it. I have tried it and you're broke 'til kingdom come. When I'm shopping, I just have to think 'filling things, filling things'.

There's not enough money to buy wholemeal bread, so I buy white bread because it's cheaper. There isn't enough money to buy cheese for them. They have orange squash instead of pure orange juice.

I try not to buy this junk food, you know. I try to give her proper food wherever possible. It's not easy. I'd like to give her more vegetables, but the vegetables are just too expensive and of course they're all pre-packed, aren't they, you can't buy them loose up here.

We used to have a proper dinner twice a week but now we have sausages and fish fingers instead. I like to make pies with real meat from the butcher, but I have to buy tinned filling now, because it's cheaper. I used to cook a big evening meal every night . . . . Now I get slices of bread to cover breakfast and sandwiches, almost exactly. I budget to the last slice of bread now.

(Graham 1985)

While an absolute definition of poverty helps us understand the constraints that shape these 'choices' about health behaviour, a relative definition pinpoints what it means to be living outside the community of which both parents and children would like to be a part. Again, the health effects are likely to be measured in psychological as well as physical terms. As one mother, living with her husband and two children on supplementary benefit observed:

We had a car but we can't afford it now. You can't afford a social life, not one where money is involved. I rarely meet people as I so rarely go out of the house. The older children go to school on their own, and, with my husband around during the day, I don't have much opportunity to go out on my own. My husband does the big shop on the bus to the shopping centre. It's too expensive for us all to go in. So it's stressful in respect of the finances. You feel inadequate in that you can't provide for the children in the way you would like – food, clothing, most things. My finances isn't enough.

(Graham 1986)

Health behaviour in poverty

The financial strategies that mothers develop in the struggle to meet health needs and avoid (too much) debt need to be set in the context not only of their housekeeping role. They need to be set, too, in the context of their health-keeping role. As health keepers, mothers provide most of the day-to-day care of children. Nearly 90 per cent of the time spent on childcare tasks in two-parent households with pre-school children is provided by mothers (Piachaud 1985).

Research suggests that poverty mediates their experiences in two major ways. First, in prioritizing fixed items, mothers cut back on other areas of consumption – food, clothes, make-up, toys, public transport, outings, playgroups – through which they and their children feel part of the world beyond the home (Burghes 1980; Graham 1986; Mayall 1986). Mothers and children in low-income households spend large proportions of their day together and alone at home, in a physical and social environment which can be less than health-promoting. Going to the shops is likely to provide the major reason to leave their immediate neighbourhood.

Second, in such circumstances, mothers tend to develop complex – and often fragile – coping strategies. These strategies typically depend on self-help: providing a way of surviving shortages of material and psychological resources alone. Although health-sustaining, these coping strategies can also be health-threatening, promoting family welfare but only by undermining individual health. In this category of coping strategies that simultaneously sustain and undermine family health, mothers often identify sweets, crisps, and biscuits for children and cigarettes for themselves.

Cigarettes are the one exception to the budgeting strategy that low income families adopt in the struggle to make ends meet. As Table 8.9 makes clear, the pattern of spending on cigarettes is similar to that of fuel and food: relative spending is higher in households with children among those on lower income. In other words, spending on tobacco 'behaves' like a necessity rather than a luxury item. Reflecting the priority that expenditure on tobacco receives in the family budget, it is often described in these terms. As one mother in the study put it:

215

I try to cut down to save money but cigarettes are my one luxury and at the moment they feel a bit like a necessity.

(Graham 1987c)

In describing why smoking is both luxury and necessity, respondents have pointed to the way in which smoking a cigarette was associated with breaks from caring: it was a way of structuring time in which, however briefly, they could rest and re-fuel. Not only was smoking associated with the maintenance of caring routines, it was also part of the way in which smokers coped with breakdowns in this routine. It was described as a way of coping when the demands of children became 'too much to cope with'. When asked what they did in these circumstances, the mothers in the study typically described how they created a space – symbolic or physical – between themselves and their children, and then filled this space with a self-directed activity. Smoking a cigarette was a major self-directed activity for mothers who smoked, as one mother explained:

If it's nice, I send them out or ask them to play in the bedroom but normally I sit in the kitchen and have a cup of coffee and a cigarette and then it's just being on my own to sort of count to ten and start again.

(Graham 1987c)

Her comments suggest that smoking a cigarette provides a way of keeping calm in situations of stress. While not designed as an analysis of caring in poverty, Brown and Harris' study of depression highlights the vulnerability of women with children caring in disadvantaged circumstances (Brown and Harris 1978). The highest rates of clinical depression were found among working-class women, without paid employment, who were caring for three or more children under five and lacked what the researchers defined as a confiding relationship with their husband/partner. One third of the women caring in these circumstances were identified as having the symptoms of clinical depression.

Depression and stress appear as part of the complex health consequences of caring in poverty: of living a lifestyle reduced to only 'what is absolutely necessary for physical health' (Rowntree 1941: 31). In such circumstances, smoking can be both necessity and luxury: a necessity that enables a woman to maintain her role as family health-keeper and a luxury that symbolizes her participation in the lifestyle of the wider society. Cigarettes offer moments when, however temporarily, the experience of relative poverty is suspended. As two mothers – one from a study by Julie Wells – explained:

> I think smoking stops me getting so irritable. I can cope with things better. If I was economising, I'd cut down on cigarettes but I wouldn't give up. I'd stop eating. . . . Food just isn't that important to me but having a cigarette is the only thing I do just for myself.
>
> (Graham 1987c)

> I'm a heavier smoker because I'm in all day. I don't go out, don't drink and don't have a car. It's the only pleasure I do have.
>
> (J. Wells 1987)

The mothers in the study explained why they spent some of their limited resources on sweets for their children in a similar way:

> If we can afford it, we do like to get them a lolly when the [ice cream] van comes round because all the kids are out there. The first week [after the two weeks' payment of benefit] and going into the second, they can have a lolly. But after that, we haven't got much money left so we can't let them have it.

> I feel I have to give them sweets sometimes as they don't get toys and clothes. They won't ever get new toys or new clothes, but I can afford 10 pence for them to buy sweets.
>
> (Graham 1986)

CONCLUSION

Health behaviour figures centrally in the current debate about the nation's health. It is seen as the common underlying factor in the major causes of death for both men and women. While a key area of health research and policy, neither the concept nor the experience of health behaviour has been subjected to systematic scrutiny in terms of its significance for women. There is an absence of feminist analysis of a concept and experience which describes what many women do on a routine basis for much of their lives.

This chapter has set out to fill this gap. By linking quantitative and qualitative data, it has sought to develop an understanding of health behaviour in terms of the wider structures that shape women's lives. In particular, it has explored women's caring role in the context of poverty, drawing on qualitative research which records women's accounts of coping with caring.

The chapter has noted how health behaviour, in research and policy, tends to be defined in an individualistic and one-dimensional way. Defined in this way, research has been able to isolate the links between individual behaviour and individual health. It has thus been possible to identify and label certain patterns of behaviour, like cigarette smoking and exercise, as either health-damaging or health-promoting. This type of research has played an important part in highlighting the role of 'lifestyle factors' in women's health in general and in the major causes of women's mortality in particular. It has pointed to the class differences in risk-taking behaviour, with cigarette smoking and poor diet, for example, concentrated among those who are most disadvantaged. Quantitative research thus points to a paradox: that it is those whose health is already at risk through the cumulative effects of social and economic disadvantage who are most likely to pursue unhealthy patterns of behaviour.

However, while a useful concept for epidemiological research, an individualistic definition of health behaviour appears to provide a less satisfactory basis for social research designed to understand why women pursue lifestyles that damage their health. Instead, we need a more complex and multi-dimensional definition of health behaviour.

As a contribution to this broader perspective on health behaviour, the chapter has explored some dimensions of women's experience of 'behaving well'. The chapter has focused on the dimensions of women's health work/health behaviour which are central to the experiences of mothers caring for children in poverty. In this context, the routines that women develop reflect a daily struggle to meet a set of *conflicting* health needs. Health-promoting behaviour includes not only behaviour that promotes individual health; health-promoting behaviour embraces, and seeks to balance, activities that protect personal health and the health of others. It embraces activities, too, which are oriented not to particular individuals but to the welfare of the household as a whole.

'Risk-taking' here takes on a specific meaning, broader and more contradictory than that found in traditional health research. Risk-taking involves patterns of behaviour which jeopardize the day-to-day economic and social survival of the family unit. Crucial to this survival is the mother's ability to manage her day-to-day responsibilities for caring within the constraints imposed by judicious housekeeping. These constraints mean that priority is given, not to food and other expenditures related directly to health, but to paying the rent and meeting financial commitments to outside agencies. In these circumstances, behaviours which damage individual health – a poor diet, cigarette smoking, sweets – can, at the same time, provide the means by which the welfare of the family is promoted. Health choices are experienced more as health compromises which, repeated day after day, become the routines which keep the family going.

In the lives of mothers living on low incomes, we can glimpse the complexity of identifying and pursuing patterns of behaviour that promote health. While the constraints are etched in sharp relief among mothers in poverty, they are likely to be ones which confront many women in their attempts to 'behave well' for themselves and for those they care for. Qualitative data can help us understand the paradoxes that quantitative data reveal. Women's accounts of their lives as health keepers can enable us to appreciate something of the responsibility of 'irresponsible' health behaviour.

REFERENCES

Abbott, P. and Sapsford, R. (1987) *Women and Social Class*, London: Tavistock.

Acker, J., Barry, K., and Esseveld, J. (1983) 'Objectivity and truth: problems in doing feminist research', *Women's Studies International Forum* 6, 4: 423–35.

Aitken-Swan, J. and Easson, E. C. (1959) 'Reactions of cancer patients on being told their diagnoses', *British Medical Journal* 1: 779-83.

Alderson, M. (1986) Letter, *British Medical Journal* 293, 23 August: 503.

Alderson, M. and Donnan, S. (1978) 'Hysterectomy rates and their influence upon mortality from carcinoma of the cervix', *Journal of Epidemiology and Community Health* 32: 175–7.

Allan, G. (1985) *Family Life: Domestic Roles and Social Organisation*, Oxford: Basil Blackwell.

Allen, S. (1982) 'Gender inequality and class formation' in A. Giddens and G. Mackenzie (eds) *Social Class and the Division of Labour*, Cambridge: Cambridge University Press.

Allin, P., Arber, S., Dale, A., and Gilbert, G. N. (1983) *Sex Differences in Sickness Absence from Work: evidence from the General Household Survey and other sources*, EOC Working Paper, Manchester: Equal Opportunities Commission (mimeo).

Altman, D. G., Gore, S. M., Gardner, M.J., and Pocock, S. J. (1983) 'Statistical guidelines for contributors to medical journals', *British Medical Journal* 286: 1489–93.

Amirikia, H. and Evans, T. N. (1979) 'Ten year review of hysterectomies: trends, indications and risk', *American Journal of Obstetrics and Gynaecology* 134: 431–7.

Antilla, S. and Isokoski, M. (1985) 'Unexpected control-group behaviour in an intervention study', *Lancet* 5 January: 43 (letter).

Arber, S. (1987) 'Social class, non-employment, and chronic illness: continuing the inequalities in health debate', *British Medical Journal* 194: 1069–73.

—— (1989) 'Gender and class inequalities in health: understanding the differentials' in A. J. Fox (ed.) *Inequalities in Health in European Countries*, Aldershot: Gower.

—— (1990) 'Opening the "Black" box: understanding inequalities in women's health', in P. Abbott and G. Payne (eds) *New Directions in the Sociology of Health*, Brighton: Falmer Press.

Arber, S. and Gilbert, G. N. (1989a) 'Transitions in caring: gender, life course and the care of the elderly', in B. Bytheway, T. Keil, P. Allatt, and A. Bryman (eds) *Becoming and Being Old: Sociological Approaches to Later Life*, London: Sage.

—— (1989b) 'Men: the forgotten carers', *Sociology* 23, 1: 111–18.

Arber, S., Gilbert, G. N., and Dale, A. (1985) 'Paid employment and women's health: a benefit or a source of role strain?', *Sociology of Health and Illness* 7, 3: 375–400.

Arber, S., Dale, A., and Gilbert, G. N. (1986) 'The limitations of existing social class classifications for women', in A. Jacoby (ed.) *The Measurement of Social Class*, London: Social Research Association.

Arber, S., Gilbert, G. N., and Evandrou, M. (1988) 'Gender, household composition and receipt of domiciliary services by elderly disabled people', *Journal of Social Policy* 17, 2: 153–75.

Ballantine, E. J. (1975) 'Objective measurements and the double-blind procedure', *American Journal of Ophthalmology* 79: 763–7.

Barker, R. and Roberts, H. (1986) 'Social classification scheme for women', *Working Paper No 51*, London: Social Statistics Research Unit, City University.

Bart, P. (1981) 'Seizing the means of reproduction: an illegal feminist abortion collective – how and why it worked', in H. Roberts (ed.) *Women, Health and Reproduction*, London: Routledge & Kegan Paul.

Benjamin, B. (1989) *Population Statistics: a review of UK sources*, Aldershot: Gower.

Beral, V. (1979) 'Reproductive mortality', *British Medical Journal* 2: 632–4.

Berkman, L. F. (1984) 'Assessing the physical health effects of social networks and support', *Review of Public Health* 413:5.

Bhat, A., Carr-Hill, R., and Ohri, S. (eds) (1988) *Britain's Black Population: a new perspective*, Aldershot: Gower.

Birke, L. (1986) *Women, Feminism and Biology*, Brighton, Sussex: Wheatsheaf Books.

Bland, M. (1987) *An Introduction to Medical Statistics*, Oxford: Oxford University Press.

Blane, D. (1985) 'An assessment of the Black Report's "explanations of health inequalities"', *Sociology of Health and Illness* 7, 3: 423–5.

Blaxter, M. (1983) 'Health services as a defence against the consequences of poverty in industrialised societies', *Social Science and Medicine* 17, 16: 1139–48.

—— (1985) 'Self-definition of health status and consulting rates in primary care', *Quarterly Journal of Social Affairs* 1, 2: 131–71.

Bone, M. (1973) *Family planning services in England and Wales*, London: HMSO.

—— (1978) *The family planning services: changes and effects*, London: HMSO.

Bone, M. and Meltzer, H. (1989) *The prevalence of disability among children*, OPCS surveys of disability in Great Britain, Report 3, London: HMSO.

Boston Women's Health Book Collective (1978) *Our Bodies Ourselves*, British edition edited by A. Phillips and J. Rakusen, Harmondsworth: Penguin.

Boyd, C. and Francome, C. (1983) *One Birth in Nine: Caesarean Section Trends since 1978*, London: Maternity Alliance.

Bracken, M. B. (1984) 'Design and conduct of randomised clinical trials in perinatal research', in M. D. Bracken (ed.) *Perinatal Epidemiology*, New York: Oxford University Press.

Bracken, M. B. (1987) 'Clinical trials and the acceptance of uncertainty', *British Medical Journal* 294: 1111–12.

Bradshaw, J. and Morgan, J. (1987) *Budgeting on Benefit: the Consumption of Families on Social Security*, London: Family Policy Studies Centre.

Brahams, D. (1983) 'Informed consent does not demand full disclosure of risks', *Lancet*, July 2: 58.

British Medical Association (1981) 'Local ethical committees', *British Medical Journal* 282: 1010.

British Medical Journal (1977) 'Hysterectomy and sterilisation – change of fashion and mind', (editorial), 2: 715–16.

—— (1986) 'Lies, damned lies and suppressed statistics', (editorial): 349–50.

Brody, H. (1977) *Placebos and the Philosophy of Medicine*, Chicago: University of Chicago Press.

Brown, C. (1984) *Black and White Britain: the Third PSI Survey*, Aldershot, Hants: Gower.

Brown, G. and Harris, T. (1978) *The Social Origins of Depression*, London: Tavistock.

Brownell, K. D. and Strunkard, A. J. (1982) 'The double blind in danger: untoward consequences of informed consent', *American Journal of Psychiatry* 139, 11: 1487–9.

Buck, N., Devlin, H. B., and Lunn, J. N. (1988) *The Report of a Confidential Enquiry into Perioperative Deaths*, London: Nuffield Provincial Hospital Trust.

Bulmer, M. (1986) *Social Science and Social Policy*, London: Allen & Unwin.

Bunker, J. P. (1970) 'Surgical manpower: a comparison of operations and surgeons in the United States and England and Wales', *New England Journal of Medicine* 285, 3: 135–44.

Bunker, J. P. and Brown, B. W. (1974) 'The physician-patient as an informed consumer of surgical services', *New England Journal of Medicine* 290: 1051–5.

Bunker, J. P., McPherson, K., and Henneman, P. L (1977) *Elective Hysterectomy Costs, Risks and Benefits of Surgery*, New York: Oxford University Press.

Burghes, L. (1980) *Living from Hand to Mouth: a Study of 65 Families Living on Supplementary Benefit*, London: Child Poverty Action Group.

Campbell, R. and Macfarlane, A. (1987) *Where to be Born? The Debate and the Evidence*, Oxford: National Perinatal Epidemiology Unit.

Campbell, R., MacDonald Davies, I., MacFarlane, A., and Beral, V. (1984) 'Home births in England and Wales, 1979: perinatal mortality according to intended place of delivery', *British Medical Journal* 289: 721–4.

Cartwright, A. (1979) *The Dignity of Labour?* London: Tavistock Publications.

—— (1983) *Health Surveys in Practice and Potential*, London: King Edwards Hospital Fund for London.

—— (1986) 'Who responds to postal questionnaires?', *Journal of Epidemiology and Community Health* 40: 267–73.

Cartwright, A. and O'Brien, M. (1976) 'Social class variations in health care and in the nature of general practitioner consultations', *Sociological Review Monograph* 22, 77–98.

Cassem, N. H. and Stewart, R. S. (1975) 'Management and care of the dying patient', *International Journal of Psychiatry in Medicine* 6: 229–38.

Central Statistical Office (annually) *Government Statistics, a Brief Guide to Sources*, London: HMSO.

—— (1986) *Guide to Official Statistics*, No. 5, London: HMSO.

—— (1989) *Social Trends* 19, London: HMSO.

Centrewall, B. S. (1981) 'Premenopausal hysterectomy and cardiovascular disease', *American Journal of Obstetrics and Gynaecology* 139: 58–61.

Chalmers, I. (1983) 'Scientific inquiry and authoritarianism in perinatal care and education', *Birth* 10, 3: 151–64.

—— (1987) Personal communication.

Chalmers, I., Campbell, H., and Turnbull, A. C. (1975) 'Use of oxytocin and incidence of neonatal jaundice', *British Medical Journal* 2: 116–18.

Chalmers, I., Zlosnik, J. E., Johns, K. A., and Campbell, H. (1976) 'Obstetric practice and outcome of pregnancy in Cardiff residents, 1965–73', *British Medical Journal* 1: 735–8.

Chalmers, I., Enkin, M., and Keirse, M. J. N. C. (1989) *Effective Care in Pregnancy and Childbirth*, Oxford: Oxford University Press.

Chamberlain, M. (1981) *Old Wives Tales*, London: Virago.

Chapman, M. (in collaboration with Basil Mahon) (1986) *Plain Figures*, London: HMSO.

Chard, T. and Richards, M. P. M. (1977) *Benefits and Hazards of the New Obstetrics*, London: Spastics International Medical Publications.

Charlesworth, A., Wilkin, D., and Durie, A. (1984) *Carers and Services: a comparison of men and women caring for dependent elderly people*, Manchester: Equal Opportunities Commission.

Cochrane, A. L (1972) *Effectiveness and Efficiency; random reflections on health services*, London: Nuffield Provincial Hospital Trust.

Cohen, S. and Syme, S. L. (1985) *Social Support and Health*, New York, Academic Press.

Coleman, L. and Dickenson, C. (1984) 'The risks of healing: the hazards of the nursing profession', in W. Charkin (ed.) *Double Exposure: Women's Health Hazards on the Job and at Home*, New York: Monthly Review Press.

Consensus Development Conference (1986) 'Treatment of primary breast cancer', *British Medical Journal* 293: 946–7.

Cornwell, J. (1984) *Hard-earned Lives: Accounts of Health and Illness from East London*, London: Tavistock.

Coronary Drug Project Research Group (1980) 'Influence of adherence to treatment and response of cholesterol on mortality in the coronary drug project', *New England Journal of Medicine* 303: 1038–41.

Coulter, A. and McPherson, K. (1986) 'The hysterectomy debate', *Quarterly Journal of Social Affairs* 2, 4: 379–93.

Coulter, A., McPherson, K., and Vessey, M. (1988) 'Do British women undergo too many or too few hysterectomies?', *Social Science and Medicine* 27, 9: 987–94.

Cox, B. *et al.* (1987) *The Health and Lifestyle Survey*, London: Health Promotion Research Trust.

Dale, A. (1986) 'Labour market participation and household dynamics', Guildford: University of Surrey (mimeo).

Dale, A., Arber, S., and Gilbert, G. N. (1982) 'Sex differences in sickness absence from work: a report based on the General Household Survey for 1975 and 1976', Report to the EOC, May, Guildford: University of Surrey (mimeo).

Dale, A., Gilbert, G. N., and Arber, S. (1985) 'Integrating women into class theory', *Sociology* 19, 3: 384–409.

Dale, A., Arber, A., and Procter, M. (1988) *Doing Secondary Analysis*, London: Unwin Hyman.

Daly, M. (1973) *Beyond God the Father*, Boston, MA: Beacon Press.

Davies, I. M. M. (1970) 'Perinatal and infant deaths: social and biological factors', *Population Trends* 19: 19–21.

Davies, K. and Esseveld, J. (1986) 'Reflections on research practices in feminist research', Paper presented at 4: e nordiska symposiet for kvinnoforskning, 11 samhallsgeografi, Uppsala, Sweden, 22–4 May.

Dawson, J. (1986) 'Randomised trials and informed consent in neonatal medicine', *British Medical Journal* 292: 1373–4.

Day, N. E. (1989) 'Screening for cancer of the cervix', *Journal of Epidemiology and Community Health* 43: 103–6.

Delphy, C. (1981) 'Women in stratification studies', in H. Roberts (ed.) *Doing Feminist Research*, London: Routledge & Kegan Paul.

Department of the Environment (1988) *Family Expenditure Survey, 1985*, London: HMSO.

Department of Health (1988) *Health and Personal Social Services Statistics for England 1988*, London: HMSO.

Department of Health and Social Security (1976a) *On the state of the public health for the year 1975*, London: HMSO.

—— (1976b) *Prevention and Health: Everybody's Business*, London: HMSO.

—— (1978) *Health and Personal Social Services Statistics for England 1978*, London: HMSO

—— (1979) *In-Patient Statistics from the Mental Health Enquiry for England 1976*, London: HMSO.

—— (1980) *Inequalities in Health* (Black Report), London: HMSO.

—— (1987) *Promoting Better Health: The Government's Programme for Improving Primary Health Care*, Cmd. 249, London: HMSO.

—— (1988a) *John Moore proposes 'health index'*, Press release 88/67, March 2.

—— (1988b) *Low Income Families: 1985*, London: DHSS.

Department of Health and Social Security, Office of Population Censuses and Surveys (1985) *Hospital Inpatient Enquiry 1983*, London, HMSO.

—— (1987a) *Hospital Inpatient Enquiry, summary tables, 1985*, Series MB4, No 26, London: HMSO.

—— (1987b) *Hospital In-patient Enquiry, main tables, 1985*, Series MB4, No 27, London: HMSO.

—— (1988) *Hospital In-Patient Enquiry, maternity tables, 1982-1985*, Series MB4, No 28, London: HMSO.

Department of Health and Social Security, Office of Population Censuses and Surveys and Welsh Office (1980) *Hospital In-patient Enquiry, maternity tables, 1973-1976*, Series MB4, No 8, London: HMSO.

Department of Health and Social Security, Welsh Office (1970) *Domiciliary midwifery and maternity bed needs: report of the sub-committee of the standing maternity and midwifery advisory committee*, London: HMSO.

Department of Health, Welsh Office, Northern Ireland Office, Scottish Office (1989) *Working for patients*, Cm 555, London: HMSO.

Dex, S. (1984) *Women's Work Histories: An Analysis of the Women and Employment Survey*, Department of Employment Research Paper No 46, London: Department of Employment.

—— (1987) *Women's Occupational Mobility; A Life Time Perspective*, London: Macmillan.

—— (1988) 'The operational aspects of social class'. Paper presented at ESRC survey methods seminar: 'A fresh look at social classification', London: The City University, 25 March.

Dickersin, K., Chan, S., Chalmers, T. C., Sachs, H. S., and Smith, H. (1987) 'Publication bias and clinical trials', *Controlled Clinical Trials* 8: 343–53.

Doll, R. and Peto, R. (1981) 'The causes of cancer', *Journal of the National Cancer Institute* 60: 1191–308.

Doyal, L. (1985) 'Women and the National Health Service', in E. Lewin and V. Olesen (eds) *Women, Health and Healing*, London: Tavistock.

Doyal, L. and Pennell, I. (1979) *The Political Economy of Health*, London: Pluto.

Doyal. L., Hunt, G., and Mellor, J. (1981) 'Your life in their hands: migrant workers in the National Health Service', *Critical Social Policy* 1, 2: 54–71.

Doyle, J. C. (1953) 'Unnecessary hysterectomy – study of 6248 operations in 35 hospitals during 1948', *Journal of the American Medical Association* January 31: 360–5.

Draper, G. (1985) 'Cervical cancer screening', *Lancet*, ii: 788.

Drife, J. O. (1989) 'The contraceptive pill and breast cancer in young women', *British Medical Journal* 298: 1269.

Dunnell, K. (1979) *Family formation 1976*, SS1080, London: HMSO.

Dyck, F., Murphy, F. A., Murphy, J. K., Road, D. A., Boyd, M. S., Osbourne, E., Vlieger, D. D., Korchinski, B., Ripley, C., Bromley, A. T., and Innes, P. B. (1977) 'Effect of surveillance on the number of hysterectomies in the Province of Saskatchewan', *New England Journal of Medicine* 296: 1326–8.

Easterday, C. L., Grimes, D. A., and Riggs, J. A. (1983) 'Hysterectomy in the United States', *Obstetrics and Gynaecology* 62, 2: 203–12.

Eddy, D. M. (1984) 'Variations in physician practice: the role of uncertainty', *Health Affairs* 3: 74–89.

Elbourne, D. (1987) 'Subjects' views about participation in randomised controlled trial', *Journal of Reproductive and Infant Psychology* 5: 3–8.

Elshtain, J. B. (1981) *Public Man, Private Woman*, Oxford: Martin Robertson.

Enkin, M. and Chalmers, I. (eds) (1982) *Effectiveness and Satisfaction in Antenatal Care*, London: Spastics International Medical Publications.

Equal Opportunities Commission (1980) *The Experiences of Caring for Elderly and Handicapped Dependants: Survey Report*, Manchester: EOC.

—— (1983) *Sickness Absence from Work. Some Interesting Facts and Figures from the Equal Opportunities Commission* Leaflet No. EOC 207. 70K/09/83, Manchester: EOC.

—— (1988) *Women and Men in Britain: a Research Profile*, Manchester: Equal Opportunities Commission.

Equal Opportunities Review (1987) *Equal Opportunities Review* 12: 10–17.

Fader, R. and Beauchamp, T. L. (1986) *A History and Theory of Informed Consent*, New York: Oxford University Press.

Farr, W. (1839) 'Letter to the Registrar General', in *The first annual report of the Registrar General for the years 1837–8*, London: HMSO.

Faulder, C. (1985) *Whose Body Is It? The Troubling Issue of Informed Consent*, London: Virago.

Finch, J. (1984) '"It's great to have someone to talk to": the ethics and politics of interviewing women', in C. Bell and H. Roberts (eds) *Social Researching: politics, problems, practice*, London: Routledge & Kegan Paul.

—— (1987) 'Family obligations and the life course', in A. Bryman, W. R. Bytheway, P. Allatt, and T. Keil (eds) *Rethinking the Life Course*, London: Macmillan.

Fischer, J. (1973) 'Is casework effective? A review', *Social Work*, January: 5–20.

Flint, C. and Poulengeris, P. (1987) *The Know Your Midwife Report* (available from Caroline Flint, 49 Peckarmans Wood, Sydenham Hill, London SE26 6RZ).

Fogelman, K. (1980) 'Smoking in pregnancy and subsequent development of the child', *Child: Care, Health and Development* 6: 233–49.

Fogelman, K. and Manor, O. (1988) 'Smoking in pregnancy and development into early adulthood', *British Medical Journal* 297: 1233–6.

Fox, A. J. and Goldblatt, P. O. (1982) *Socio-demographic mortality differentials: longitudinal study 1971-75*, LS No. 1, London: HMSO

Fox, A. J., Goldblatt, P. O., and Adelstein, A. M. (1982a) 'Selection and mortality differentials' *Journal of Epidemiology and Community Health* 36, 2: 69–79.

Fox, A. J., Gee, D., Jones, D., and Leon, D. (1982b) *Cancer and Work: making sense of workers' experience*, London City University: Statistical Laboratory and General and Municipal Workers Union.

Fox, A. J., Goldblatt, P. O. and Jones, D. R. (1985) 'Social class mortality differentials: artefact, selection or life circumstances', *Journal of Epidemiology and Community Health* 39, 1: 1–8.

Freeman, R. (1989) Written parliamentary reply, House of Commons Official Report (Hansard), March 6, col 415.

Freidson, E. F. (1970) *Professional Dominance: the social structure of medical care*, Chicago: Aldine.

Garcia, J. (1982) 'Women's views of antenatal care', in M. Enkin and I. Chalmers (eds) *Effectiveness and Satisfaction in Antenatal Care*, London: Spastics International Medical Publications.

Gath, D., Cooper, P., and Day, A. (1982) 'Hysterectomy and psychiatric disease I: Levels of psychiatric morbidity before and after hysterectomy', *British Journal of Psychiatry* 40: 335–50.

General Register Office (1923) *Census of England and Wales, 1911, Volume XIII, Part II*, London: HMSO.

—— (1938) *Registrar General's Decennial Supplement on occupational mortality, 1931, England and Wales, Part II, Occupational mortality*, London: HMSO.

Gillon, R. (1987) *Philosophical Medical Ethics*, Chichester: John Wiley.

Glendinning, C. and Millar, J. (1987) 'Invisible women, invisible poverty', in C. Glendinning and J. Millar (eds) *Women and Poverty in Britain*, Brighton, Sussex: Wheatsheaf Books.

—— (eds) (1987) *Women and Poverty in Britain*, Brighton: Wheatsheaf Books.

Goffman, E. (1968) *Stigma: Notes on the management of spoiled identity*, Harmondsworth: Penguin.

Goldblatt, P. (ed.) (forthcoming) 'Mortality and social organisation', LS No. 6, London: HMSO.

Goldthorpe, J. H. (1983) 'Women and class analysis: in defence of the conventional view', *Sociology* 18, 4: 465–88.

—— (1984) 'Women and class analysis: a reply to the replies', *Sociology* 18, 4: 497–9.

Gore, S. (1988) 'The quality of life in a clinical context' (Report of ESRC workshop on measuring the quality of health), *Survey Methods Newsletter* Winter, London: Social and Community Planning Research.

Gore, S. M. and Altman, D. G. (1982) *Statistics in Practice*, London: British Medical Association Press.

Government Statisticians Collective (1979) 'How official statistics are produced: views from the inside', in J. Irvine, I. Miles, and J. Evans (eds) *Demystifying Official Statistics*, London: Pluto.

Grafe, W. R., McSherry, C. K., Finkel, M. C., and McCarthy, E. G. (1978) 'The elective surgery second opinion programme', *Annals of Surgery* 188: 323–30.

Graham, H. (1984) *Women, Health and the Family*, Brighton: Wheatsheaf Books.

—— (1985) *Caring for the Family* (Full Report), Milton Keynes: Open University.

—— (1986) *Caring for the Family*, Research Report No. 1, Milton Keynes: Open University.

—— (1987a) 'Being poor: perceptions and coping strategies of lone mothers', in J. Brannen and G. Wilson (eds) *Give and Take in Families: Studies in Resource Distribution*, London: Allen & Unwin.

—— (1987b) 'Women's poverty and caring' in C. Glendinning and J. Millar (eds) *Women and Poverty in Britain*, Brighton, Sussex: Wheatsheaf Books.

—— (1987c) 'Women's smoking and family health', *Social Science and Medicine* 25, 1: 47–56.

—— (1988) 'Women's smoking in the United Kingdom: the implications for health promotion', *Health Promotion*, 3, 4: 371–82.

Graham, H. and Oakley, A. (1981) 'Competing ideologies of reproduction: medical and maternal perspectives on pregnancy and birth', in H. Roberts (ed.) *Women, Health and Reproduction*, London: Routledge & Kegan Paul.

Grant, J. M. and Hussein, I. Y. (1984) 'An audit of abdominal hysterectomy over a decade in a district hospital', *British Journal of Obstetrics and Gynaecology* 91: 73–7.

Green, H. (1988) *Informal Carers*, OPCS, Series GHS, No 15, Supplement A, London: HMSO.

Greenwood, M. (1928) 'Contribution to the discussion on Dr Stevenson's paper', *Journal of the Royal Statistical Society* 91: 221–30.

Grimsley, M. and Bhat, A. (1988) 'Health', in A. Bhat, R. Carr-Hill, and S. Ohri (eds) *Britain's Black Population: A New Perspective*, Aldershot, Hants: Gower.

Grunder, T. M. (1980) 'On the readability of surgical consent forms', *New England Journal of Medicine* 17 April: 900–2.

Hadley, R. (1987) 'Publish and be ignored; proselytize and be damned', in G. C. Wenger (ed.) *The Research Relationship: Practice and Politics in Social Policy Research*, London: Allen & Unwin.

Hakim, C. (1982) *Secondary Analysis in Social Research*, London: Allen & Unwin.

Harding, N. (1989) 'The use and abuse of women in the NHS', *Radical Community Medicine* 37: 6–10.

Harding, S. (1986) *The Science Question in Feminism*, Milton Keynes: Open University Press.

Harris, A. I. (1971) *Handicapped and impaired in Great Britain*, SS418, London: HMSO.

Harris, H. (1974) *Prenatal Diagnosis and Selective Abortion* The Rock-Carling Fellowship, London: Nuffield Provincial Hospitals Trust.

Hedges, L. V. (1987) 'How hard is hard science? How soft is soft science?' *American Psychologist* May: 443–5.

Henwood, M. and Wicks, M. (1985) 'Community care, family trends and social change', *Quarterly Journal of Social Affairs* 1, 4: 357–71.

Herxheimer, A. (1988) 'The rights of the patient in clinical research', *The Lancet*, Nov 12: 1128–30.

Hey, E. (1980) 'Retrolental fibroplasia as one index of perinatally acquired handicaps', in I. Chalmers and G. McIlwaine (eds) *Perinatal Audit and Surveillance*, London: Royal College of Obstetrics and Gynaecology.

Holmes, H. (1988) 'Low income families in Tyne and Wear'. *Cash and Care* 4: 2, York: University of York.

Homans, H. (1983) 'A question of balance: Asian and British women's perception of food during pregnancy', in A. Murcott (ed.) *The Sociology of Food and Eating*, Aldershot, Hants: Gower.

—— (1989) *Women in the National Health Service*, London: HMSO.

Homer, M., Leonard, A., and Taylor, P. (1984) *Private Violence: Public Shame*, Middlesbrough, Cleveland: Cleveland Refuge and Aid for Women and Children.

Huff, D. (1973) *How to Lie with Statistics*, Harmondsworth: Pelican.

Hunt, A. (1986) 'Use of quantitative methods in researching issues which affect women', *Methodological Issues in Gender Research*, EOC Research Bulletin No 10: 12–19, Manchester: Equal Opportunities Commission.

Hutton, S. (1986) 'Low income families and fuel debt', in I. Ramsey (ed.) *Debtors and Creditors*, London: Professional Books.

Hyde, S., Balloch, S., and Ainley, P. (1989) *A Social Atlas of Poverty in Lewisham*, London: Centre for Inner City Studies, Goldsmith's College.

Hyman, H. H. (1972) *Secondary Analysis of Sample Surveys*, New York: Wiley.

Interdepartmental Committee on Physical Deterioration (1904) *Report*, Cd 2175, London: HMSO.

Irvine, J., Miles, I., and Evans, J. (eds) (1979) *Demystifying Social Statistics*, London: Pluto Press.

Johnson, A. and King, R. (1990) 'A regional register of early childhood impairments: a discussion paper', *Community Medicine* (in press).

Joshi, H. (1986) 'Participation in paid work: evidence from the Women and Employment Survey', in R. Blundell and I. Walker (eds) *Unemployment, Search and Labour Supply*, Cambridge: Cambridge University Press.

Jowell, R., Witherspoon, S., and Brook, L. (1988) *British Social Attitudes: the 5th Report*, Aldershot, Hants: Gower.

Keller, E. F. (1982) 'Feminism and science', *Signs: Journal of Women in Culture and Society* 7, 3: 589–602.

Kiernan, K. (1988) 'Who remains celibate?, *Journal of Biosocial Science* 20: 253–63.

King, J. (1986) 'Informed consent', *Bulletin of the Institute of Medical Ethics*, Supplement No 3, December.

Klein, R. and Rowland, R. (1989) 'Hormonal cocktails: women as test-sites for fertility drugs', *Women's Studies International Forum* 12: 333–48.

Laing, A. H., Berry, R. J., Newman, C. R., and Peto, J. (1975) 'Treatment of inoperable carcinoma of bronchus', *Lancet* 13 December: 1161–4.

Land, H. (1978) 'Who cares for the family?', *Journal of Social Policy* 7, 3: 257–84.

Laurance, J. (1986) 'How Ministers fiddle figures' (Society in Focus), *New Society* 76 (Feb 28): 362.

Lewis, C. E. (1969) 'Variation in the incidence of surgery', *New England Journal of Medicine* 281: 880–4.

Lewis, J. and Meredith, B. (1988) *Daughters Who Care: Daughters Caring for Mothers at Home*, London: Routledge.

Lockwood, E. (1971) 'Accuracy of Scottish morbidity data', *British Journal of Preventive Medicine* 25: 76–83.

Loft, A., Andersen, T. F., and Madsen, M. (1986) 'Regional variations in hysterectomy in Denmark', *International Newsletter on Regional Variations in Health Care* 2: 2.

Loftus, E. F. and Fries, J. F. (1979) 'Informed consent may be hazardous to health', *Science* 204: 11.

Lumley, J. (1989) Personal communication.

Lumley, J., Lester, A., Renon, P., and Wood, C. (1985) 'A failed RCT to determine the best method of delivery for very low birthweight infants', *Controlled Clinical Trials* 6: 120–7.

McCord, J. (1981) 'Consideration of some effects of a counselling programme', in S. E. Martin, L. B. Sechrest, and R. Redner (eds) *New Directions in the Rehabilitation of Criminal Offenders*, Washington: National Academy Press.

—— (1982) 'The Cambridge-Somerville Youth Study: a sobering lesson on treatment, prevention and evaluation', in A. J. McSweeny, W. J. Freeman, and R. Hawkins (eds) *Practical Program Evaluation in Youth*, Springfield, Illinois: Charles C. Thomas.

McCormick, A. (1988) 'Trends in mortality statistics in England and Wales with particular reference to AIDS from 1984 to April 1987', *British Medical Journal* 296: 1289–92.

McDowall, M. E. (1983) 'Measuring women's occupational mortality', *Population Trends* 34: 25–9.

—— (1985) *Occupational reproductive mortality*, Studies on Medical and Population Subjects No 50, London: HMSO.

Macfarlane, A. J. (1980) 'Official statistics and women's health and illness', *EOC Research Bulletin No 4:* 43–77, Manchester: Equal Opportunities Commission.

—— (1988a) 'The downs and ups of infant mortality', *British Medical Journal* 296: 230–1.

—— (1988b) 'Holding back the tide of caesareans', *British Medical Journal* 297: 852.

Macfarlane, A. J. and Mugford, M. (1984) *Birth Counts: Statistics of Pregnancy and Childbirth*, London: HMSO.

McIntosh, J. (1976) 'Patients' awareness and desire for information about diagnosed but undisclosed malignant disease', *Lancet* 7: 300–3.

Macintyre, S. (1976) 'To have or have not – promotion and prevention in gynaecological work', in M. Stacey (ed.) *The Sociology of the NHS*, Sociological Review Monograph 22, Staffordshire: University of Keele.

McKee, L. (1987) 'Households during unemployment: the resourcefulness of the unemployed', in J. Brannen and G. Wilson (eds) (1987) *Give and Take in Families: Studies in Resource Distribution*, London: Allen & Unwin.

McKeigue, P., Marmot, M., Adelstein, A., Hunt, S., Shipley, M., Butler, S., Riemersma, R., and Turner, P. (1985) 'Diet and risk factors for coronary heart disease in Asians in north-west London', *Lancet* 8464: 1086–90.

McPherson, K. (1989) 'Cervical cytology policy', *Lancet* ii: 162–3.

McPherson, K., Strong, P. M., Epstein, A., and Jones, L. (1981) 'Regional variations in the use of common surgical procedures: within and between England and Wales, Canada and the United States', *Social Science and Medicine* 15A: 273–88.

McPherson, K., Wennberg, J. E., Hovind, O. B., and Clifford, P. (1982) 'Small area variations in the use of common surgical procedures: an international comparison of New England, England and Norway', *New England Journal of Medicine* 307: 1310–14.

Madge, N. and Marmot, M. (1987) 'Psychosocial factors and health', *The Quarterly Journal of Social Affairs* 3, 2: 81–134.

Marmot, M. (1986) 'Social inequalities in mortality: the social environment', in R. Wilkinson (ed.) *Class and Health: Research and Longitudinal Data*, London: Tavistock.

Marmot, M. and McDowall, M. (1986) 'Mortality decline and widening social inequalities', *Lancet*, ii: 274–6.

Marmot, M., Adelstein, A., and Bulusu, L. (1984) *Immigrant Mortality in*

REFERENCES

England and Wales 1970–78, OPCS Studies on Medical and Population Subjects, No 47, London: HMSO.

Marsh, A. and Matheson, J. (1983) *Smoking Attitudes and Behaviour*, London: HMSO.

Marsh, C. (1988) *Exploring Data: An Introduction to Data Analysis for Social Scientists*, Cambridge and Oxford: Polity Press in association with Basil Blackwell.

Martin, C. J. (1987a) 'Monitoring maternity services by postal questionnaire: congruity between mothers' reports and their obstetric records', *Statistics in Medicine* 6: 613–27.

—— (1987b) 'Responding to public need: a study of housing and health', *Radical Community Medicine* 30: 28–34.

Martin, J. and Roberts, C. (1984) *Women and Employment: A Lifetime Perspective*, Department of Employment/OPCS, London: HMSO.

Martin, J., Meltzer, H., and Elliot, D. (1988) *The prevalence of disability among adults*, OPCS surveys of disability in Great Britain, Report 1, London: HMSO.

Mason, V. (1989) *Women's Experience of Maternity Care – A Survey Manual*, London: HMSO.

Mattson M. E., Curb, J. D., McArdle, R., and the AMIS & BHAT Research GPs (1985) 'Participation in a clinical trial: the patient's point of view', *Controlled Clinical Trials* 6: 156–67.

Mayall, B. (1986) *Keeping Children Healthy*, London: Allen & Unwin.

Micklethwait, P., Jenkins, C. C., Flanagan, G. L., Mansfield, R., Beech, B., Wynn, A., and Wynn, M. (1982) Letter to the *Observer* 25 July.

Miles, I. and Irvine, J. (1979) 'The critique of official statistics', in J. Irvine, I. Miles, and J. Evans (eds) *Demystifying Official Statistics*, London: Pluto.

Miller, N. (1946) 'Hysterectomy: therapeutic necessity or surgical racket?', *American Journal of Obstetrics and Gynaecology* 51: 804–10.

Millman, M. and Kanter, R. M. (eds) (1975) *Another Voice: Feminist Perspectives on Social Life and Social Science*, New York: Anchor Books.

Mitchell, J. (1984) *What is to be done about illness and health? Crisis in the eighties*, Harmondsworth: Penguin.

Moser, K. and Goldblatt, P. (1990) 'Occupational mortality of women aged 15–59 at death', *Working Paper No. 66*, London: Social Statistics Research Unit, City University.

Moser, K., Pugh, H., and Goldblatt, P. (1988a) 'Inequalities in women's health: looking at mortality differentials using an alternative approach', *British Medical Journal* 296: 1221–4.

—— (1988b) 'Inequalities in women's health in England and Wales: mortality among married women according to social circumstances, employment characteristics and life cycle stage', *Working Paper No. 57*, London: Social Statistics Research Unit, City University.

New Society (1978) 'His equals hers', June 15, 44(819): 584.

Newton, T. (1988) Written parliamentary reply, House of Commons Official report, (Hansard), April 13.

Nicholl, J. P., Thomas, K. J., William, B. T., and Knowelden, J. (1984) 'Contribution of the private sector to elective surgery in England and Wales', *Lancet* July 14: 89–92.

Nicholl, J. P., Beeby, N. R., and Williams, B. T. (1989a) 'Comparison of the activity of short stay independent hospitals in England and Wales, 1981 and 1986', *British Medical Journal* 298: 239–42.

—— (1989b) 'Role of the private sector in elective surgery in England and Wales, 1986', *British Medical Journal* 298: 243–7.

Nichols, T. (1979) 'Social class: official, sociological and marxist', in J. Irvine, I. Miles, and J. Evans (eds) *Demystifying Social Statistics*, London: Pluto.

Nissel, M. (1980) 'Women in government statistics: basic concepts and assumptions', *Equal Opportunities Commission Research Bulletin* 4: 5–28.

—— (1984) 'The family costs of looking after handicapped elderly relatives', *Ageing and Society* 4, 2: 185–205.

—— (1987) *People Count*, London, HMSO.

Nissel, M. and Bonnerjea, L. (1982) *Family Care of the Handicapped Elderly: Who Pays?*, London: Policy Studies Institute.

Nobel, A. D. (1985) 'Management of menorrhagia', *British Medical Journal* 291: 296–7.

Oakley, A. (1974) *Housewife*, London: Allen Lane.

—— (1979) *Becoming a Mother*, Oxford: Martin Robertson.

—— (1981) 'Interviewing women: a contradiction in terms?', in H. Roberts (ed.) *Doing Feminist Research*, London: Routledge & Kegan Paul.

—— (1984) *The Captured Womb*, Oxford: Blackwell.

—— (1985) 'Social support in pregnancy: the "soft" way to increase birthweight?', *Social Science and Medicine* 21, 11: 1259–68.

—— (1988) 'Is social support good for the health of mothers and babies?', *Journal of Infant and Reproductive Psychology* 6: 3–21.

—— (1990) 'Who's afraid of the randomized controlled trial? Some dilemmas of the scientific method and "good" research practice', *Women and Health* 15, 2.

Oakley, A. and Oakley, R. (1979) 'Sexism in official statistics', in J. Irvine, I. Miles, and J. Evans (eds) *Demystifying Social Statistics*, London: Pluto Press.

Oakley, A., McPherson, A., and Roberts, M. (1990) *Miscarriage*, Harmondsworth: Penguin.

O'Brien, M. (1978) 'Home and hospital: a comparison of the experiences of mothers having home and hospital confinements', *Journal of the Royal College of General Practitioners* 28: 460–6.

Office of Health Economics (1981) *Sickness Absence – A Review*, Briefing No 16, London: Office of Health Economics.

Office of Population Censuses and Surveys (1965–84) 'Hysterectomy rates in England and Wales', *Ad hoc* information request.

—— (1978a) *Occupational mortality 1970–72. The Registrar General's Decennial Supplement for England and Wales*, (Series DS No 1), London: HMSO.

—— (1978b) *General Household Survey 1976*, London: HMSO

—— (1978c) *Mortality Statistics, Cause 1976, England and Wales* Series DH2, No. 3, London: HMSO.

—— (1979) *General Household Survey 1977*, London: HMSO.

—— (1980) *General Household Survey 1978*, Series GHS No 8, London: HMSO.

—— (1982) *General Household Survey, 1980*, London: HMSO.

—— (1984a) *General Household Survey, 1982*, London: HMSO.

—— (1984b) *Census 1981, Household and Family Composition, England and Wales*, CEN 81 HFC, London: HMSO.

—— (1985a) *Birthweight Statistics 1984*, OPCS monitor DH3 85/6, London: HMSO.

—— (1985b) *General Household Survey 1983*, Series GHS No. 13, London: HMSO.

—— (1986a) *Occupational Mortality: The Registrar General's Decennial Supplement for Great Britain, 1979–80, 1982–83*, Series DS No 6, London: HMSO.

—— (1986b) *General Household Survey 1984*, Series GHS No 14, London: HMSO.

—— (1986c) *Birth Statistics 1985*, Series FM1 No 12, London: HMSO.

—— (1987) *General Household Survey 1985*, Series GHS No 15, London: HMSO.

—— (1988a) *Registration: a modern service. Proposals to reform the system for registering births, marriages and deaths in England and Wales*, Cm 531, London: HMSO.

—— (1988b) *Cancer registration 1984*, Series MB1, No 16, London: HMSO.

—— (1988c) *The Longitudinal Study* (1971–81) CEN81 LS, London: HMSO.

—— (1988d) *Informal Carers: General Household Survey 1985*, London: HMSO.

—— (1988e) *Mortality statistics, cause, 1986, England and Wales*, Series DH2 No 13, London: HMSO.

—— (1989a) *General Household Survey 1986*, Series GHS No 16, London: HMSO.

—— (1989b) *Legal abortion 1988*, OPCS Monitor AB 89/3, London: OPCS.

—— (1989c) *Mortality statistics, 1986, England and Wales*, Series DH1 No 18, London: HMSO.

—— (1989d) *Mortality statistics, accidents and violence, 1986, England and Wales*, Series DH4 No 12, London: HMSO.

Ohri, S. and Faruqi, S. (1988) 'Racism, employment and unemployment', in A. Bhat, R. Carr-Hill, and S. Ohri (eds) *Britain's Black Population: a New Perspective*, Aldershot, Hants: Gower.

Open University (1985) 'Hysterectomy: a surgical epidemic?' *Health and Disease*, U205, book 11: 59–71.

Pahl, J. (1988) 'Earning, sharing, spending: married couples and their money', in R. Walker and G. Parker (eds) *Money Matters: Income, Wealth and Financial Welfare*, London: Sage.

Papaioannou, A. (1982) 'Informed consent after randomisation', Letter, *Lancet* 9 October: 828.

Parker, G (1985) *With due care and attention, a review of research on informal care*, Occasional Paper No 2, London: Family Policy Studies Centre.

—— (1988) 'Indebtedness', in R. Walker and G. Parker (eds) *Money Matters: Income, Wealth and Financial Welfare*, London: Sage.

Patel, A. P., Gray, G., Lang, G. D., Baillie, F. G. H., Fleming, F., and Wilson, G. M. (1976) 'Scottish hospital morbidity data: errors in diagnostic returns', *Health Bulletin* 34: 215–20.

Payne, J. (1987) 'Does unemployment run in families? Some findings from the General Household Survey', *Sociology* 21, 2: 199–214.

Perry, B. W. (1976) 'Time trends in hysterectomy 1970-1975', *PAS Reporter* 14: 9.

Peters, D. and Ceci, S. (1982) 'Peer-review practices of psychology journals: the fate of published articles submitted again', *The Behavioural and Brain Sciences* 5: 187–255.

Piachaud, D. (1985) *Round About Fifty Hours a Week: The Time Costs of Children*, London: Child Poverty Action Group.

Pill, R. and Stott, N. (1985) 'Preventive procedures and practices among working-class women: new data and fresh insights', *Social Science and Medicine* 21, 9: 975–83.

Pinder, C. D. (1982) 'Catchment populations: the properties and accuracy of various methods for their estimation', *Community Medicine* 4: 188–95.

Pokras, R. and Hufnagel, V. G. (1988) 'Hysterectomy in the United States 1965–1984', *American Journal of Public Health* 78, 7: 852–3.

Popay, J. and Jones, G. (1988) 'Gender inequalities in health: explaining the sting in the tail', paper presented to the Social Policy Association Annual conference, July, University of Edinburgh.

Pugh, H., Power, C., Goldblatt, P., and Arber, S. (1989) 'Smoking, class and lung cancer mortality among women in England and Wales',

Working Paper No 63, London: Social Statistics Research Unit, City University.

Radical Statistics Health Group (1981) *The Unofficial Guide to Official Health Statistics*, second edition (new edition in preparation), London: Radical Statistics.

—— (1987) *Facing the Figures: what really is happening to the National Health Service?*, London: Radical Statistics.

Rapoport, R. M. (ed.) (1985) *Children, Youth and Families – the Action-Research Relationship*, Cambridge: Cambridge University Press.

Reinharz, S. (1981) 'Experimental analysis: a contribution to feminist research', in G. Bowler and R. Duelli-Klein (eds) *Theories of Women's Studies: II*, Berkeley, California: University of Berkeley, Women's Studies Department.

Richards, D. H. (1973) 'Depression after hysterectomy', *Lancet* ii: 430–2.

—— (1974) 'A post-hysterectomy syndrome', *Lancet* ii: 983–5.

Roberts, H. (ed.) (1981) *Doing Feminist Research*, London: Routledge & Kegan Paul.

—— (1984) 'Putting the show on the road: the dissemination of research findings', in C. Bell and H. Roberts (eds) *Social Researching: Politics, Problems, Practice*, London: Routledge & Kegan Paul.

—— (1985) *The Patient Patients*, London: Pandora.

Roberts, H. and Barker, R. (1987) *What are People Doing when They Grade Women's Work?*, LS Working Paper No 52, London: Social Statistics Research Unit.

Robinson, J. (1987) 'Cervical cancer – doctors hide the truth?' in S. O. Sullivan (ed.) *Woman's Health: A Spare Rib Reader*, London: Pandora Press.

Roman, E., Beral, V., and Inskip, H. (1985) 'Occupational mortality among women in England and Wales', *British Medical Journal* 291: 194–6.

Roos, N. P. (1984a) 'Hysterectomies in one Canadian province. A new look at risks and benefits', *American Journal of Public Health* 74, 1: 39–46.

—— (1984b) 'Hysterectomy: variations in rates across small areas and across physicians' practice', *American Journal of Public Health* 74, 4: 327–35.

Rose, H. (1983) 'Hand, brain and heart: a feminist epistemology for the natural sciences', *Signs: Journal of Women in Culture and Society* 9(11): 73–90.

Rose, H. and Rose, S. (1979) 'Radical science and its enemies', in R. Miliband and J. Saville (eds) *Socialist Register*, Atlantic Highlands, N J: Humanities Press.

Rowbotham, S. (1985) 'What do women want? Women-centred values and the world as it is', *Feminist Review* 20: 49–69.

Rowntree, B. S. (1902) *Poverty: A Study of Town Life*, London: Macmillan.
—— (1941) *Poverty and Progress*, London: Longman.
Royal College of General Practitioners, Office of Population Censuses and Surveys, Department of Health and Social Security (1979) *Mortality statistics from general practice: second national survey*, 1970–1, Studies on Medical and Population Subjects, No. 26, London: HMSO.
—— (1986) *Mortality statistics from general practice 1981–2: third national survey*, Series MB5 No 1, London: HMSO.
Royal College of Physicians (1983) *Smoking or Health*, London; Pitman Educational.
Rutkow, I. M. (1982) 'Unnecessary surgery? What is it?' *Surgical Clinics of North America* 621: 613–25.
Ruzek, S. B. (1978) *The Women's Health Movement*, New York: Praeger.
Sandberg, S. I., Barnes, B. A., Weinstein, M. C., and Brain, P. (1983) 'Elective hysterectomy. Benefits, risks and cost', *Medical Care* 23, 9: 1067–85.
Schacht, P. J. and Pemberton, A. (1985) 'What is unnecessary surgery? Who shall decide? Issues of consumer sovereignty, conflict and self-regulation', *Social Science and Medicine* 20, 3: 199–206.
Schwarz, D., Flamant, R., and Lellouch, J. (1980) *Clinical Trials*, London: Academic Press.
Scotsman (1989) Report of Nicholas Ridley's address to the Association of Metropolitan Authorities, Newcastle-upon-Tyne (10/7/89), *The Scotsman* 11 July: 4.
Scottish Health Statistics (1988) Information and Statistical Division, Common Services Agency, Edinburgh.
Scottish Morbidity Records 1 (1961-84) SMR1, Information and Statistics Division, Common Services Agency.
Selman, S. F. (1988) *Family Planning. Review of UK statistical sources, Vol XXV*, London: Chapman & Hall.
Selwood, T. and Wood, C. (1978) 'Incidence of hysterectomy in Australia', *Medical Journal of Australia* 2: 201–4.
Shaper, A., Pocock, S., Walker, M., Phillips, A. N., Whitehead, T. P., and Macfarlane, P. W. (1985) 'Risk factors for ischaemic heart disease: the prospective phase of the British Regional Heart Study', *Journal of Epidemiology and Community Health* 39: 197–209.
Sherman, J. A. and Beck, E. T. (1979) (eds) *The Prism of Sex: essays on the sociology of knowledge*, Madison, WI: University of Wisconsin Press.
Silverman, W. A. (1980) *Retrolental Fibroplasia: a modern parable*, New York: Grune & Stratton.
—— (1985) *Human Experimentation: a guided step into the unknown*, Oxford: Oxford University Press.

Simes, R. J., Tattersall, M. H. N., Coates, A. S., Radhavan, D., Solomon, H. J., and Smart, H. (1986) 'Randomised comparison of procedures for obtaining informed consent in clinical trials and treatment for cancer', *British Medical Journal* 293: 1065–8.

Smith, A. and Jacobson, B. (eds) (1988) *The Nation's Health*, London: King Edward's Hospital Fund for London.

Smith, A., Elkind, A., and Eardley, A. (1989) 'Making cervical cancer screening work', *British Medical Journal* 298: 1662–4.

Smith, D. (1975) 'Women and mental health statistics', in D. Smith and S. David (eds) *Women Look at Psychiatry*, Vancouver BC: Press Gang.

Smith, D. E. (1979) 'A sociology for women', in J. A. Sherman and E. T. Beck (eds) *The Prism of Sex: essays on the sociology of knowledge*, Madison, WI: University of Wisconsin Press.

Smith, H. D. T. (1981) 'Analysis of the accuracy of the data recorded on SMR1', Glasgow: Greater Glasgow Health Board.

Spallone, P. and Steinberg, D. L. (eds) (1987) *Made to Order: the myth of reproductive and genetic progress*, Oxford: Pergamon Press.

Stanworth, M. (1984) 'Women and class analysis: a reply to John Goldthorpe', *Sociology* 18, 2: 159–70.

Steering Group on Health Services Information (1985) Supplement to the First and Fourth Reports to the Secretary of State, London: HMSO

Stevenson, T. H. C. (1910) 'Suggested lines of advance in English vital statistics', *Journal of the Royal Statistical Society* 53: 685–709.

—— (1927) 'Occupational mortality, fertility and infant mortality', in *The Registrar General's Decennial Supplement for England and Wales, Part II*, London: HMSO.

—— (1928) 'Vital statistics of wealth and poverty', *Journal of the Royal Statistical Society* 91: 207–30.

Studd, J. (1989) 'Prophylactic oophorectomy', *British Journal of Obstetrics and Gynaecology* 96, 5: 506–9.

Tatham, J. (1908) 'Letter to the Registrar General on high mortality in certain occupations in the three years 1900, 1901, 1902', in *Supplement to the 65th annual report of the Registrar General, Part II*, London: HMSO.

Terry, P., Condie, R., and Settatree, R. (1980) 'Analysis of ethnic differences in perinatal statistics', *British Medical Journal* 281: 1307.

Tew, M. (1981) 'Effects of scientific obstetrics on perinatal mortality', *Health and Social Services Journal* 91: 444–6.

Thomas, E. (1988) 'How doctors secret trials abused me', *The Observer*, October 9: 12.

Titmuss, R. M. (1970) *The Gift Relationship*, London: Allen & Unwin.

Todd, J. E. and Walker, A. M. (1980) *Adult dental health, Volume 1, England and Wales, 1968-78*, SS1112, London: HMSO.

Todd, J. E. and Dodd, T. (1985) *Children's dental health in the United Kingdom, 1983*, SS1189, London: HMSO.

Todd, J. E., Walker, A. M., and Dodd, P. (1982) *Adult dental health, Volume 2, United Kingdom 1978*, SS1112, London: HMSO.

Townsend, P. (1979) *Poverty in the United Kingdom*, Harmondsworth: Penguin.

—— (1987) *Poverty and Labour in London*, London: Low Pay Unit.

Townsend, P., Davidson, N., and Whitehead, M. (1988) *Inequalities in Health: the Black Report and the Health Divide*, Harmondsworth: Penguin.

Traub, A. I., Thompson, W., and Gibson, L. (1980) 'Hysterectomy in young women – a thirty year review', *British Journal of Clinical Practice* 34, 89: 233–7.

Ungerson, C. (1987) *Policy is Personal; Sex, Gender and Informal Care*, London: Tavistock.

Vayda, E. and Anderson, G. D. (1975) 'Comparison of provincial surgical rates in 1968', *Canadian Journal of Surgery* 18: 18–26.

Veit-Wilson, J. (1986) 'Paradigms of poverty: a rehabilitation of B. S. Rowntree', *Journal of Social Policy* 15, 1: 69–99.

Waitzkin, H. and Streckle, J. (1976) 'Information control and the micropolitics of health care: summary of original research project', *Social Science and Medicine* 10: 263–76.

Walker, A. M. and Jick, H. (1979) 'Temporal and regional variation in hysterectomy rates in the United States 1970–1975', *American Journal of Epidemiology* 110, 1: 41–6.

Webb, J. (1986) (personal communication, Community Medicine Specialist) Information Services Division, Common Services Agency, Edinburgh.

Weber, M. (1919) 'Politics as a vocation', in H. H. Gerth and C. Wright Mills (eds and trans.) *From Max Weber: Essays in Sociology*, London: Routledge & Kegan Paul, 1970.

Wells, J. (1987) *Women and Smoking: an evaluation of the role of stress in smoking cessation and relapse*, Southampton: Department of Psychology, University of Southampton.

Wells, N. (1987) *Women's Health Today*, London: Office of Health Economics.

—— (1989) 'The health of Britain's women', in Medical Women's Federation *Women, Health and Work*, Proceedings of the Medical Women's Federation 70th Annual Symposium, London: Medical Women's Federation.

Wenger, G. C. (1987) 'Establishing a dialogue', in G. C. Wenger (ed.) *The Research Relationship: Practice and Politics in Social Policy Research*, London: Allen & Unwin.

Wennberg, J. E. (1984) 'Dealing with medical practice variations: a proposal for action', *Health Affairs* 3: 6–32.

Wennberg, J. E. and Gittelsohn, A. (1973) 'Small area variations in health care delivery. A population based health information system can guide planning and regulating decision making', *Science* 182: 1102–8.

Wertz, R. W. and Wertz, D. C. (1977) *Lying-In: a history of childbirth in America*, Glencoe: The Free Press.

Wheeler, E. and Tan, S. P. (1983) 'Food for equilibrium: the dietary principles and practice of Chinese families in London' in A. Murcott (ed.) *The Sociology of Food and Eating*, Aldershot, Hants: Gower.

Wijma, K., Kauer, F. M., and Janssens, J. (1984) 'Indication for, prevalence and implications of hysterectomy: a discussion', *Journal of Psychosomatic Obstetrics and Gynaecology* 3: 69–77.

Wilkinson, R. (1986) 'Socio-economic differences in mortality: interpreting the data on their size and trends', in R. Wilkinson (ed.) *Class and Health: Research and Longitudinal Data*, London: Tavistock.

Wingo, P. A., Huezo, C. M., Rubin, G. L., Ory, H. W., and Peterson, H. B. (1985) 'The mortality risk associated with hysterectomy', *American Journal of Obstetrics and Gynaecology* 152: 803–8.

Wood, S. (1988) 'IVF woman in coma', *The Sun* (Melbourne Australia), March 3.

World Health Organisation (1986) *Having a Baby in Europe*, European Regional Office, Copenhagen.

Wright, F. (1983) 'Single carers: employment, housework and caring' in J. Finch and D. Groves (eds) *A Labour of Love: Women, Work and Caring*, London: Routledge & Kegan Paul.

Wright, R. (1969) 'Hysterectomy: past, present and future' (Editorial), *Obstetrics and Gynaecology* 33, 4: 560–3.

Zelen, M. (1979) 'A new design for randomised clinical trials', *New England Journal of Medicine* 31 May: 1242–5.

NAME INDEX

SUBJECT INDEX

Note: As women's health is the subject of this book, there are no index entries under 'women'; the reader is advised to seek more specific references. Men's health is indexed under 'gender differences'.